THE
HEALTHY
BACK
DIRECTORY

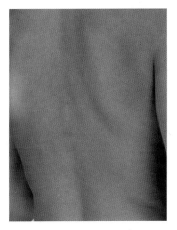

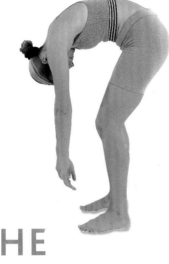

THE
HEALTHY
BACK
DIRECTORY

a complete guide to caring for your back, bones, joints and muscles

KIM DAVIS
consultant editor *Dr. Anthony Campbell*

METRO BOOKS
NEW YORK

This 2009 edition published by Metro Books,
by arrangement with Ivy Press.

Note from the publisher
This book should be considered as a reference source only and it is not intended to replace instruction or advice from a qualified practitioner or other healthcare professional. The author and publisher disclaim any liability, loss, injury, or damage incurred as a consequence, directly or indirectly, of the use and application of the contents.

This book was conceived, designed, and produced by
Ivy Press
The Old Candlemakers
West Street, Lewes, East Sussex, BN7 2NZ, UK

Creative Director PETER BRIDGEWATER
Publisher SOPHIE COLLINS
Editorial Director JASON HOOK
Design Manager SIMON GOGGIN
Designer JANE LANAWAY
Senior Project Editor REBECCA SARACENO
Editor MANDY GREENFIELD
Studio Photography GUY RYECART
Picture Librarian SHARON DORTENZIO
Illustrations MICHAEL COURTNEY, GUY SMITH

Metro Books
122 Fifth Avenue
New York, NY 10011

ISBN-13: 978-1-4351-0883-7
ISBN-10: 1-4351-0883-3

Originated and printed in China

1 3 5 7 9 10 8 6 4 2

Contents

A Healthier Life

Back pain is the most common of the aches and ailments to which we are all prone. More than 90 percent of people suffer from back problems at one time or another, and for many it is a recurring or constant fact of life.

This book shows you how to go about protecting your back, bones, and joints, and offers ways of dealing with troubles when they occur. By paying attention to your posture, and by making some simple adjustments to the way you drive, work, eat, and exercise, you can ensure that you are placing minimal strain on your body's infrastructure.

The book is divided into sections, each of which deals with a particular aspect of the body—your back, your bones, your joints, and your muscles. Each chapter includes a

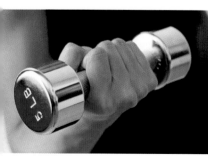
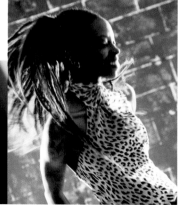

reference section, which explains the most common diseases and injuries to affect that part of the body and advises you when you should consult a doctor.

The directory contains advice on dealing with problems such as sciatica, arthritis, and sports injuries. It covers remedial exercises, suggestions for self-treatment, and complementary therapies that may help. A final section looks at how aging affects us—and shows you some techniques that could help you live a longer, stronger, more active life.

The Directory of Your Back, Your Bones & Things That Ache aims to put you in touch with all the information you need to take control of your well-being and to keep yourself healthy and pain-free.

Regular exercise is an important aspect of maintaining good health —but it is important that you choose the right form of exercise for you. This book helps you to decide, and includes specific exercises to help common problems.

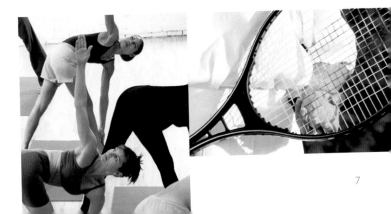

The Skeleton

Our bones form the tough framework that gives the body its shape and strength. The skeleton enables us to stand upright, to move, and to pick things up. It also provides protection for the vulnerable internal organs—the heart and lungs, for example, are surrounded by the tough bars of the ribcage.

Our bones are living tissues, which are constantly being renewed. They are made up of collagen and minerals. Collagen gives bones their shock-absorbing abilities, while minerals such as calcium, phosphorus, and magnesium make them strong.

Inside your bones

The bones are not solid: inside the dense outer layer is a honeycomb-like scaffolding of spongy bone. This makes our bones strong but light—so that they can support us, without weighing us down. Inside the bone is bone marrow, a fatty substance that makes our red blood cells.

❶ Periosteum

❷ Spongy bone

❸ Compact bone

❹ Artery and vein

❺ Bone marrow

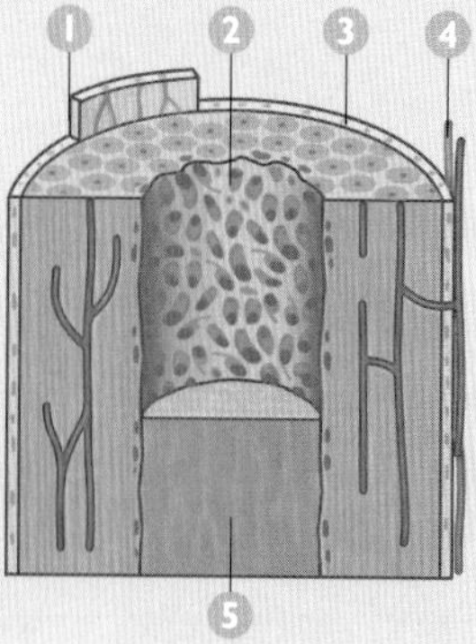

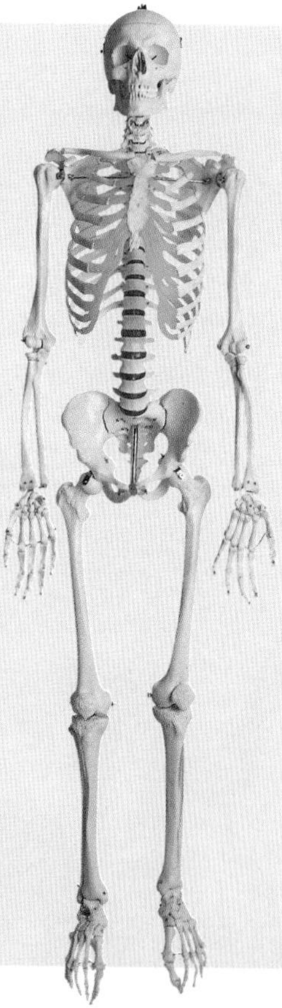

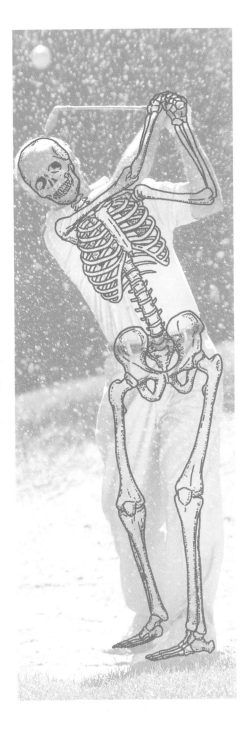

Types of bones

The bones are ingeniously designed to perform a variety of functions in the body.

1 Long bones The arms and legs have long bones. These act as levers and can be used for moving the body.

2 Short bones The box-like bones of the wrists and ankles have greater strength than long bones, but still let limited movement take place.

3 Flat bones The bones of the skull are flat, to create a protective casing for the brain. The shoulder blades are other examples of flat bones in the body.

4 Irregular bones Certain bones have distinctive shapes that help them to support particular parts of the body: the bones of the spine, for instance, fit together to encircle the entire length of the spinal cord. Irregular bones are also found in the pelvis, hips, and face.

Left: **Our bones work in conjunction with our muscular system, letting us maintain an upright position and move.**

The Spine

There are 33 irregularly shaped bones in the spine. These vertebrae are connected to each other by tiny joints, which allow movement and give the spine stability. Between the vertebrae are disks of cartilage, which act as shock absorbers. Two large ligaments run down the spine, and smaller ones connect the vertebrae. These and the muscles of the back help control our spinal movements.

The vertebrae have slightly different shapes depending on where they are. The seven vertebrae of the neck (the cervical spine) are smaller than the others, allowing greater movement. The upper thoracic spine consists of 12 vertebrae; these have extra joints to which the ribs are attached. The five vertebrae of the lumbar spine are large and sturdy, because this area bears most of our body weight. The sacrum consists of five vertebrae fused together; the coccyx (tailbone) of four vertebrae, also joined together.

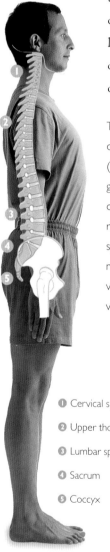

❶ Cervical spine

❷ Upper thoracic spine

❸ Lumbar spine

❹ Sacrum

❺ Coccyx

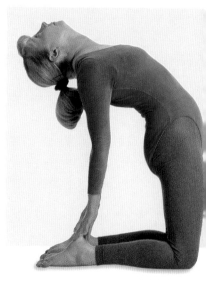

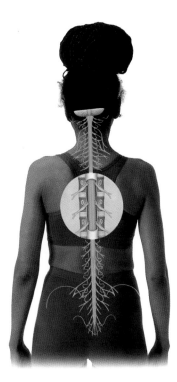

The spinal cord

The spinal cord is an information highway between the brain and the body. It runs down a channel in the bones of the upper spine, which form a protective casing around it. Nerves branch off the spinal cord and pass through gaps in the vertebrae. Both the spinal nerves and the spinal cord are vulnerable to damage if the spine is injured.

Moving around

A healthy, flexible spine should be able to bend backward and forward and twist from side to side.

Most of the movement comes from the lower back and the neck—the ribs attached to the thoracic spine prevent it from bending to the side. Regular exercise helps to maintain mobility in the spine.

The Joints

Joints are the hinges between two or more bones. In most joints the bones fit loosely together, letting movement take place easily: these are known as synovial joints. Other joints, called semimovable joints, allow less movement but provide stability: they include the joints of the spine and pelvis. The joints of the skull are fixed: the bones are tightly fitted together to form a protective casing for the brain.

Types of joint

Shown right are all the joint types found in the body. There are six types of synovial (movable) joint. They are classified according to the shape of the bones, how they fit together, and the range of movement allowed.

❶ **Fixed** The bones of the skull are connected by tough, fibrous tissue that permits no movement to take place. The skull contains the only fixed joints in the body.

❷ **Semimovable** In these joints, the bones are connected to a disk of cartilage, which allows only limited movement. The pelvic and spinal bones are semimovable joints.

❸ **Pivot** In this joint, one bone forms a collar while the other rotates within it. Pivot joints are found in the neck, letting the head turn from side to side, and in the forearms.

❹ **Hinge** One bone fits into the groove of another, allowing a bending or straightening action. The knee and elbow are hinge joints.

❺ **Ellipsoid** One bone forms an oval cup-shape into which the oval end of the other bone fits, as in the wrist. This allows movement in all directions, including some rotation.

❻ **Ball and socket** This type of joint permits movement in all directions. The end of one bone forms a ball-shape and fits into a rounded socket formed by the other. The hip and shoulder are ball-and-socket joints.

❼ **Saddle** Two bones meet at right angles, allowing up–down and sideways movement. The thumb is the body's only saddle joint.

❽ **Gliding/plane** This type of joint lets bones slide over each other. Plane joints are found in the feet and hands.

Inside a synovial joint

The ends of the bones in a synovial joint, such as the knee, are covered in slippery cartilage. This helps to minimize friction and allow smooth movement. The bone ends also receive constant lubrication from the synovial fluid, which is secreted by the joint lining. Strong ligaments stabilize and support the joint.

❾ Patella

❿ Synovial fluid

⓫ Patellar tendon (ligament)

⓬ Articular cartilage

⓭ Joint capsule

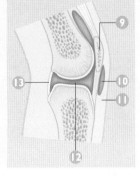

The Muscular System

There are more than 650 muscles in the human body. Together they make up about 40 percent of our body weight. Muscles power our movements and enable us to maintain postures such as standing or holding up an arm. All muscles work in the same way: by contracting and relaxing. There are two main types of muscle. Voluntary or skeletal muscles are those that we can move at will—for example, the muscles of the legs. They are attached to our bones by bands of strong fibrous tissue (tendons). Involuntary muscles are those over which we exercise no control. They include the muscles inside our blood vessels, the heart, and other internal organs.

Inside your muscles

A skeletal muscle is made up of many bundles (fascicles) of strong, thread-like fibers, which are surrounded by a sheet of connective tissue. Each fiber consists of tiny threads called myofibrils, which contain thick and thin strands of filament. When stimulated by a nerve impulse, the filaments slide closer together, causing the myofibrils and, ultimately, the muscle to contract.

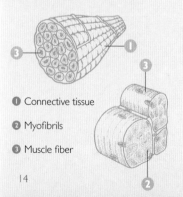

❶ Connective tissue

❷ Myofibrils

❸ Muscle fiber

All muscles are able to contract (shorten) and relax (lengthen). In the human body, muscles and bones work together in pairs, and when one muscle contracts, its partner relaxes. When a muscle contracts, it pulls the bone to which it is attached toward the anchor point. When it relaxes, and its partner contracts, the bone is pulled in the opposite direction. This dual action is what enables movement to take place. The muscles of the back, which are situated in layers, work in conjunction with the abdominal muscles to give the spine stability and to permit a wide range of movement without strain.

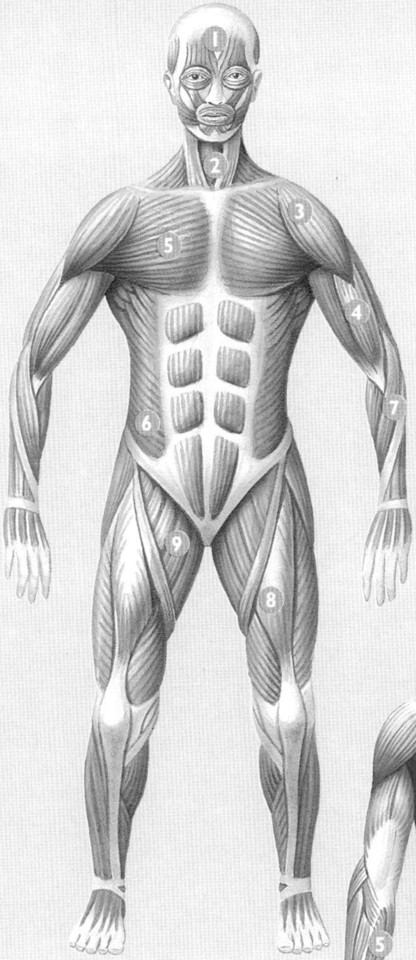

Front of body

❶ Face muscles

❷ Neck muscles

❸ Deltoid

❹ Biceps

❺ Chest muscles

❻ Abdominal muscles

❼ Extensors of wrist and fingers

❽ Quadricep muscles

❾ Groin muscles

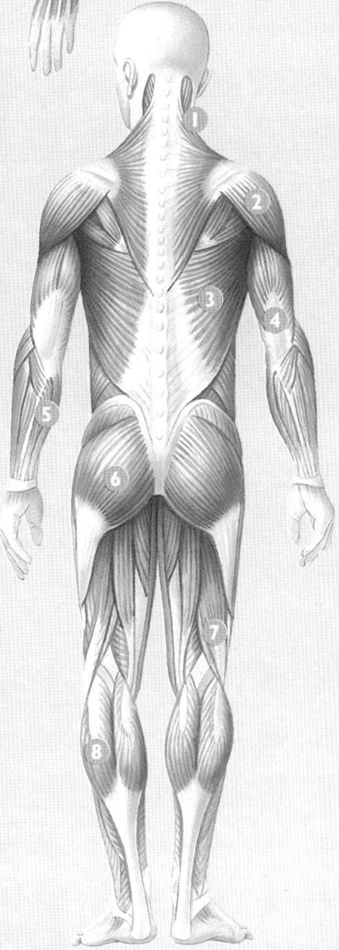

Back of body

❶ Neck muscles

❷ Deltoid

❸ Back muscles

❹ Triceps

❺ Extensors of wrist and fingers

❻ Gluteus maximus

❼ Hamstring muscles

❽ Calf muscles

How We Move

Muscles, bones, and joints work together to generate movement. As we have seen, muscles are attached to bones at the joints by means of tendons. But muscles can only pull; they cannot push. For this reason, they tend to be arranged in pairs, one on each side of a joint. One muscle relaxes as the other contracts, to hoist the bone into position.

To lift up your forearm, for example, you tighten the biceps in the top of your arm. It becomes shorter and fatter, pulling the bones in your forearm upward. At the same time, the triceps muscle on the underside of your arm relaxes. To lower the forearm, the triceps muscle tightens, while the biceps relaxes and lengthens.

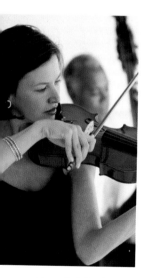

Above: A violin player has her arm continually bent at the elbow as she plays, meaning that her biceps is contracted and her triceps relaxed.

Bending and straightening the arm

The simple action of bending and straightening the arm offers a classic example of muscles at work, with the biceps and triceps counter-balancing each other and operating in tandem.

❶ Biceps contracting

❷ Triceps relaxing

❸ Biceps relaxing

❹ Triceps contracting

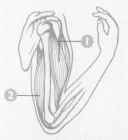

Your Back

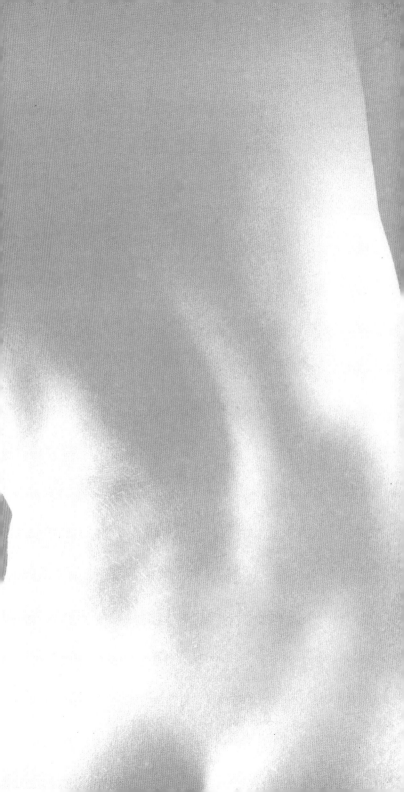

Your Posture

Children have naturally good posture, and they instinctively move in a way that places minimum strain on the body, but most people develop poor postural habits as they grow up. We may tense the shoulders, slouch when we sit, or stand with most of our weight pushed onto one leg. Over time, these bad habits place the body under pressure and can lead to pain and long-term damage. Learning to stand, sit, and move correctly helps to protect the back from harm.

Posture pointers

Be aware of your spine whenever you are standing. Imagine that an invisible cord is attached to the top of your head, helping to lift you into an erect, relaxed posture. These tips should help ensure that you stand correctly.

① Head Keep your head erect and in line with the spine. Your chin should be level with the floor, and your neck free from tension.

② Shoulders Your shoulders should remain relaxed and level. Draw your shoulder blades in and down the back.

③ Pelvis Keep your hips level. Tuck your tailbone slightly inward to help support the spine.

④ Knees Always maintain a slight bend in your knees—they need to be soft, not locked.

⑤ Feet Keep your weight equally balanced between both feet.

Positioning your pelvis

Many people have a tendency to tilt the pelvis too far backward or forward, which throws the spine out of alignment. Try sitting or kneeling to practice the correct position.

Correct position

Here the pelvis is correctly aligned with the spine. The tailbone is tucked in and the sitting bones extend down to the floor, as the hips lift upward slightly.

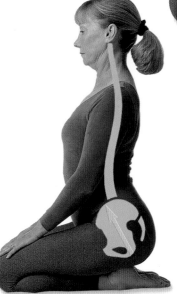

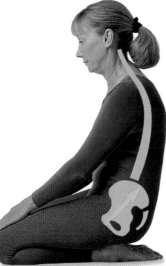

Pelvis tilting forward

Here the pelvis is tilted forward and the tailbone is pushed backward. This puts pressure on the abdominal and lower back muscles.

Pelvis tilting backward

Here the tailbone is drawn too far inward, with the result that the pelvis tips backward. This strains the lower back and distorts the curve of the upper back.

Basic Back Care

Most back problems are the result of poor posture or sudden strain on the muscles. They can often be prevented by becoming more aware of your movements and posture. The following are some simple ways to help protect your back from the general stresses and strains of daily life.

Always sit in an upright position, keeping both feet flat on the floor.

Developing postural awareness

Most of us do not notice when we are standing or sitting badly, but it is easy to develop greater postural awareness. At frequent intervals during the day, simply stop what you are doing and check how you are holding yourself. Notice any tension or discomfort, and shift your position to relieve it. Take a few deep breaths at the same time: this helps you to relax the body before you return to whatever you are doing. Eventually you will start to notice when you are putting your body under strain and will automatically shift your position.

It will help if you practice good standing and sitting techniques for a few minutes each day—use the tips on the previous page. You should also avoid holding one position for a long time.

Avoiding strain

Many back injuries occur when the muscles are put under sudden pressure—for example, when you engage in a strenuous activity such as digging without first warming up the muscles. Before embarking on household or garden chores, try walking briskly on the spot and doing a few stretches. Avoid stooping as you work;

squat or kneel instead, and use long-handled tools wherever possible. Take frequent rests.

Never try to lift something that is too heavy for you—ask someone else to help. To lift a heavy item from the floor, stand in front of it in a wide stance. Get as close to it as possible. Squat down and take a firm hold of the base. Straighten your knees to stand up, bringing the item toward you. Lean forward slightly, but keep your back straight. Avoid twisting around or bending forward when you are carrying a heavy item.

In general, avoid carrying shopping or other loads in one bag; divide the weight equally between two bags, so that you can carry one in each hand or over each shoulder. Better still, use a backpack.

Keeping comfortable

At night, make sure that you have a comfortable mattress to sleep on: it should be firm enough to support the back without feeling too hard. Do not use too many pillows, as these twist the neck.

Women should avoid wearing high heels, which can easily push the spine out of alignment. Wear comfortable shoes, ideally with a low heel.

Lifting

To lift a heavy box, squat down and grasp the base. Straighten the legs to stand up, and bring the item toward your body.

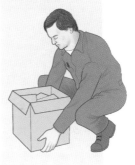

Sleep easy

Use a pillow to help keep your spine straight. Push the pillow into your shoulder to support the neck, or use a neck pillow.

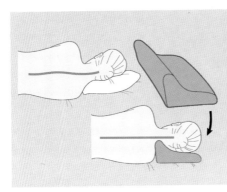

At Work and in the Car

People who sit down all day—particularly those who spend long periods at a computer or in a car—are especially prone to backache. Take the time to adjust your work station or car seat so that it offers maximum support, and take regular time out to stretch the body and realign the spine.

Below: **Adjust an office chair to make sure that it supports your spine, and is at the correct height in relation to your desk.**

If you spend hours at a computer, it is important that you adjust your work station to suit your height. The position of your desk in relation to your chair is critical—if it is too high or too low, you may develop neck and shoulder problems. Adjust

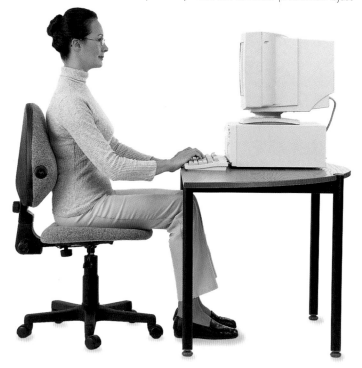

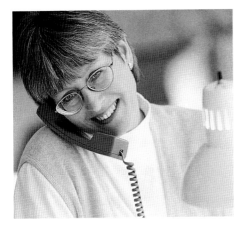

your chair so that your forearms are parallel to the floor when you type. Your elbows should be slightly lower than the forearms, and at an angle of 90° to the upper arms. Place your computer on a support: the top of the screen should be level with your eyes. Make sure that you can place your feet flat on the floor; if you can't, use a footrest.

Adjust the back of the chair so that your spine is supported. Ideally, the chair back will move with you, so that it stays in contact with your spine. Sit well back in the chair, and do not slump; keep the head and spine erect, as if they are being lifted by a cord attached to the top of your head.

Do not tuck the telephone between your neck and shoulder, because this puts unnecessary pressure on your neck. Hold the handset, or use a hands-free headset.

Above: **If you are on the phone for long periods, use a headset. Never cradle the phone under your ear, as this puts pressure on the neck.**

Tips for drivers

Adjusting your car seat will help you maintain a comfortable position. Follow these tips to protect your back.

❶ **Head** Make sure that the back of your head is supported by the head restraint. This helps to protect you from whiplash in the event of an accident.

❷ **Lower back** Adjust the seat to give maximum support to the lower back —use a cushion, a rolled-up towel, or a lumbar roll for extra comfort. Sit well back in the seat, and keep your tailbone tucked in.

❸ **Arms** Check that you can reach the wheel comfortably—your arms should be slightly bent.

❹ **Legs** Adjust the height of the seat so that you can operate the pedals easily. Move the back of the seat to increase the angle between thighs and trunk.

❺ **Relax** Whenever you come to a stop—at traffic lights, say—relax your grip on the steering wheel. Shrug your shoulders to release tension.

23

Back Exercises for the Office

Even the best position starts to feel uncomfortable if you stay in it for too long. If you work sitting down, stand up every 30 minutes or so: walk around or simply stretch out. Try doing the following exercises two or three times a day, to help release tension from the back. Sit upright, with your chin and tailbone tucked in, and work slowly, breathing normally all the time.

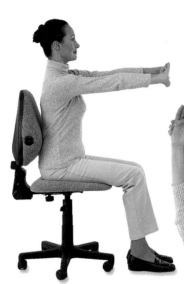

2 Vertical Arm Stretch Lift your arms over your head, placing the back of one hand in the palm of the other. Keep your arms comfortably bent. Slowly bend to the right, until you can feel a slight stretch down your left side. Return to the center and repeat on the left. Do three or four bends in each direction.

Horizontal Arm Stretch Slide your chair away from your desk, so that you have room to stretch out. Gently clasp your hands together, then raise your arms to shoulder height. Inhale and extend them fully, turning your palms outward. Exhale and lower your arms. Repeat the stretch three or four times.

3 Forward Bend Move to the front of your seat. Tighten your abdominal muscles and drop your head. Bend forward slowly, starting at the base of the neck and working all the way down the spine. Let your arms hang down. Hold for a few moments, then unfold from the base of the spine upward. Lift the head last.

4 Side Twist Sit back in the chair. Tighten your abdominal muscles, then turn slowly to the left, placing both hands on the back of the chair, as shown. Use your right hand as a lever to help increase the turn—but take care not to force the twist. Hold for a few moments, then return to the center and repeat on the other side. Do this once more.

5 Knee Bend Keeping your abdominal muscles tight, lift your right knee. Gently grasp the top of your shin with both hands. Draw the knee slowly toward you and hold for a few moments, breathing normally. Release and repeat on the left leg. Repeat twice more on each side.

6 Pelvic Rolling Draw your chair into the desk. Roll your sitting bones backward, so that the arch in your lower back is exaggerated. Then flatten the back by rolling them forward. Do this back–forward movement three or four times. Finish by sitting tall, with your tailbone tucked in. You can practice this exercise unobtrusively at any time.

Building Flexibility and Strength

Suppleness and strength are key to maintaining a healthy back. Regular exercise can improve the flexibility of the spine as well as strengthen the muscles that support it. It will also help you to shed any excess weight: being overweight can cause you to hold yourself in an awkward, and potentially harmful, way.

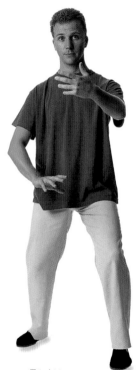

Tai chi is a very gentle form of exercise that can enhance your general posture and build strength and flexibility.

Maintaining your general fitness encourages good health and is an essential element of back care. Exercise helps to improve mobility in the joints, including those of the spine. It strengthens the muscles, which can help the trunk to cope better with load-bearing. And it improves the circulation, aiding the distribution of oxygen and nutrients to all areas of the body.

Regular exercise is also the best way in which to release the muscular tension that is one of the main causes of poor posture and backache. In addition, physical activity burns calories and thereby helps to you to lose excess weight, which may be placing an unnecessary strain on your muscles and joints.

Be sure to choose a form of exercise that is commensurate with your level of fitness and your weight. It is a good idea to take specialized advice on this—see your doctor before starting a new fitness program, particularly if you are overweight, ill, or in pain, or if you have not exercised for some time. The most gentle forms of exercise are swimming, walking, cycling, and tai chi. Walking and

Swimming: the right stroke

Swimming is a great form of exercise, so long as you use a good technique.

Doing breaststroke with your head out of the water, for instance, pushes the back out of alignment, so it may do you more harm than good. Practicing backstroke or crawl may be more beneficial.

tai chi are recommended for people of all ages, since they place minimum strain on the body.

It is important to start gently and increase your fitness slowly. Many people make the mistake of enthusiastically overexercising when they start, which can cause serious damage. If you are walking, say, start with ten minutes' walking a day and build up over several weeks to 30 minutes (depending on your fitness level). In general, most people benefit from three 30-minute sessions of moderate exercise a week.

It is a good idea to do specific back exercises in addition to following a general fitness program. A general routine is described on the following pages. Yoga and Pilates also offer excellent ways of exercising the back, but you will need an experienced teacher to guide you.

Yoga is a good way to strengthen the back and improve its flexibility.

Simple Back Routine

Ideally, you should practice gentle back exercises every day. However, if you have previously experienced back pain or problems, check their suitability with your doctor first. Always work very gently and do not force the back farther than feels natural—over time, your flexibility will increase. If you feel any pain, stop and seek advice from a doctor.

Before you begin

Wear loose, comfortable clothing, that does not restrict your movements. Warm up first: walk briskly on the spot for at least five minutes. Raise your knees a few times as you continue to walk, then swing your arms gently from side to side. When your breathing has quickened and you are feeling warm, you can start.

I   Stand tall, with your feet hip-distance apart and tailbone and chin tucked in. Bend forward, starting from the base of the neck and gradually working down the back—contract your abdominal muscles to control the movement. Hold for a few moments, then uncurl slowly from the base of your spine. Bring the head up last.

> **HELPFUL HINT**
> Run through the posture pointers on page 18 before you start each stretch. Be sure to keep your tailbone tucked in, so that your spine remains erect.

2 From an upright position, slowly turn your right shoulder to the right, letting the rest of the upper body follow the movement. Keep the head in line with the spine, and turn only as far as is comfortable. Use your abdominals to control your movement and breathe steadily. Now slowly turn back to the center, then turn to the left.

3 Starting from the upright position, extend the spine upward—as though it is being pulled up by a cord—and very gently arch it backward at the same time. Take care not to stretch farther than is comfortable, and keep your abdominal muscles tight. Keep the tailbone tucked in and your hips level. Do not throw the head back.

4 Again starting from the upright position, raise your shoulders up high, inhaling deeply as you do so. Hold for a moment, then exhale as you let them drop down gently. Do this two or three times. Make sure that your posture remains erect and relaxed at all times.

Hip Shunt and Knee Bend

Hip Shunts help to improve flexibility in the lower back and hips. You need to keep your upper body as still as possible as you move your hips. Knee Bends are a great form of exercise for releasing tension in the back. They are useful to do at any time when you are experiencing discomfort. You need a non-slip mat in order to do all the floor exercises.

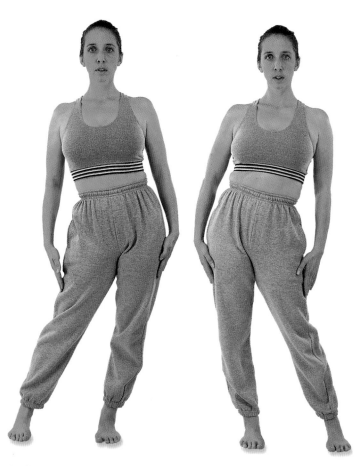

1 Stand up tall, arms by your sides, knees slightly bent, hips level. Shift your weight onto the left leg as you shunt the left hip outward. Keep the upper body still.

2 Return to the upright position and repeat on the right side. Do alternate sides several times, to make one slow, continuous movement.

1 Lie down, with your body straight and your knees bent so that you can put your feet flat on the mat—they should be hip-distance apart. Lift up the legs and bring them toward the chest, contracting your abdominal muscles to control the movement. Hold your knees with your hands—if this feels uncomfortable, place your hands below the knees on the thighs.

2 Breathing out, use your hands to pull your knees closer into the chest. You should feel a slight stretch in the lower back, but do not go farther than feels comfortable. Hold for a few moments, breathing normally, then release. Repeat two or three times.

HELPFUL HINT

When you lie down, move the sitting bones slightly upward and forward to flatten the back slightly.

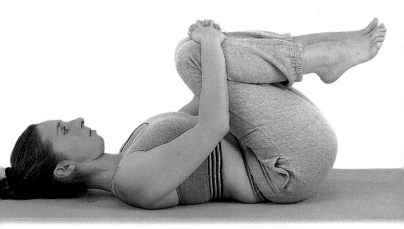

Roll to the Side

This is another good exercise to increase flexibility in the lower back. However, it is vital that you keep the movement controlled and slow, by contracting your abdominals. Never force your knees farther toward the floor than they will naturally go. If you feel any discomfort when practicing lumbar rolls, stop the exercise and do some Knee Bends (see *page 31*) to release tension in the lower back.

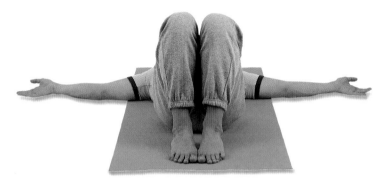

1 Lie on the mat, making sure that your body is straight. Bring your knees up so that you can rest your feet flat on the mat—your knees should be touching. Bring your arms straight out to the sides, keeping the shoulders relaxed and level. Bring the sitting bones forward and upward so that the lower back flattens slightly.

2 Now, very slowly, move your knees out to the left and toward the mat, letting your right foot and buttock rise off the mat. Go as far as you need to in order to feel a gentle stretch in the hips and lower back—you should not feel any strain. Breathe deeply for a few moments in this position.

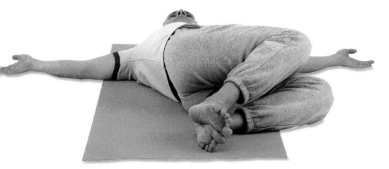

3 As you gain greater flexibility in the lower back, you will find that you can go farther each time. Eventually, you may be able to bring your knees down to the floor without discomfort, as shown here. Rest in this position for a few moments, keeping your abdominal muscles tight and continuing to breathe deeply.

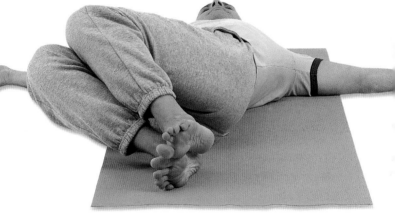

HELPFUL HINTS

It is important to keep breathing deeply throughout all the exercises. Here, you may find it helps to exhale as you roll the knees to the floor, and inhale as you bring them up again.

Many people find they are able to bring one knee closer to the floor than the other; do not try to equalize the stretch by forcing the movement on one side.

4 Very slowly bring your knees up to the center and rest your feet flat on the mat again. Make sure that your sitting bones are still in the correct position. Now roll over to the right. Repeat steps 2–4 four or five times.

Kneeling Back Arch and Forward Bend

The Kneeling Back Arch is an excellent exercise for increasing flexibility in the lower back and releasing tension in the neck and shoulders. Yoga practitioners call it the Cat, because it mimics the graceful action of that animal when it arches its back. Do not try to arch your back too far—all you need to feel is a gentle stretch in order to receive the benefit. This can also be a good exercise for women suffering from period pains.

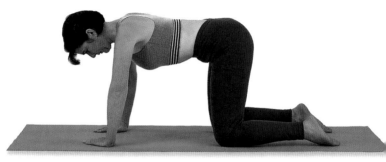

I   Kneel on all fours, with your knees hip-distance apart and your hands directly underneath your shoulders. Your fingers should point slightly inward, and your feet should point straight back. Face downward, so that your head, neck, and back are in line with each other and parallel with the floor. Contract your abdominal muscles slightly.

HELPFUL HINT

Watch that you do not lock your elbows at any point—you need to keep them slightly bent (soft) throughout the exercise.

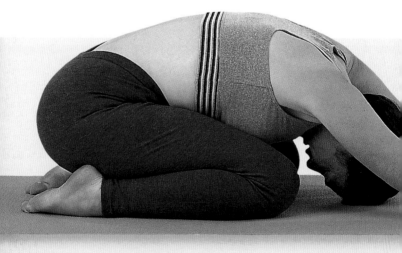

2 Breathing in, tilt your sitting bones upward so that your abdomen moves closer to the floor and your back hollows. Do not tense your shoulders or force your back into an excessive arch. Hold this position for a few moments, breathing normally.

3 Breathing out, bring your sitting bones down and arch the back upward, lifting the spine as far as feels comfortable. Drop your head between your arms, but do not bend the elbows. Hold for a few moments as you continue to breathe. Repeat steps 2 and 3 four or five times.

Forward Bend

After you have done the Back Arch, relax in this Forward Bend.

Sit back, resting your buttocks on your heels. Bend forward, dropping your forehead onto the mat. Gently stretch your arms forward, placing your hands and wrists flat on the mat. Breathe slowly and steadily in this position for a few minutes.

35

Twists, Upward Stretch, and Relaxation

Gentle Spinal Twists help to improve the back's ability to turn from side to side. You can do them sitting either on the floor or on a chair. If you are fairly stiff, do the chair-based variation for a few weeks, or until you have built up greater flexibility. Continue the routine with an Upward Stretch, to tone the muscles of the lower back. Always end a back session a minimum of five minutes' relaxation.

Spinal Twist

1 Sit upright, legs stretched out. Draw in your abdomen. Bend your right knee and place your right foot outside the left calf. Place your left elbow on the right knee, resting the hand on the thigh; place your right hand behind you. Turn to the right, lifting up from the tailbone so that the whole spine is engaged. Keep the right shoulder back.

2 Slowly return to the central position, and change your legs and hands around. Slowly turn to the left, keeping your left shoulder back. Hold and breathe. Repeat steps 1 and 2 four or five times. Keep your shoulders relaxed throughout the exercise.

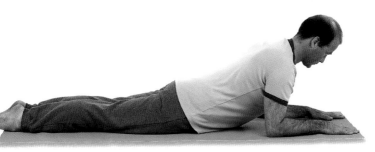

Upward Stretch

Lie down, legs together, hands in front of your head and elbows bent. Rest your forehead on the mat. Contract your abdominals. Inhale and slowly raise the upper body, extending the spine forward and keeping your tailbone in. Go only as far as feels comfortable. Hold, breathing normally, then lower yourself on an out-breath. Repeat four or five times. End with some Knee Bends (see page 31).

Relaxation

Lie on your back, and bend your knees so that your feet are flat on the floor. Tuck a pillow under your head. Your arms can either be by your sides, elbows slightly bent, or crossed over your chest, as shown. Close your eyes and breathe deeply for a few minutes. As you breathe, try to relax each area of your body in turn: your face, neck, shoulders, chest, arms, abdomen, hips, thighs, calves, feet. Let each part of you relax into the floor. To get up, roll onto your side and use your arms to lever yourself up.

Twist Variation

This chair exercise is good if you find it hard to sit on the floor.

Sit upright, feet flat on the ground. Place the right hand on the left knee, and hold the chair back with the left hand. Very gently turn to the left, lifting up from the base of the spine. Return to the center and twist to the other side. Do not turn too far. Repeat four or five times.

Build Your Strength

When you are familiar with the Simple Back Routine, try adding the strengthening exercises on these and the following pages. They should be done after the Upward Stretch on page 37 and before the Relaxation. Build your routine slowly, adding a few additional exercises at a time. Check the suitability of these exercises with your doctor if you have had back problems or any pain, or if you are ill or overweight. Stop immediately if you experience pain, and seek advice. Always respect the limitations of your own body.

Leg Lift

I Lie on your front and bend your arms so that you can rest your chin on your forearms. Stretch your legs out behind you, feet together. Tuck in your tailbone and contract your stomach muscles to give additional support to the spine. Breathe normally.

HELPFUL HINT

Make sure you do not arch the back when you lift up the leg. Keep breathing throughout the exercise, and work very slowly and with control. If you feel any pain, stop and do some Knee Bends (see page 31).

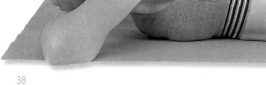

Double Leg Lift Lie with your arms by your sides, palms up and your face resting on the mat. Contract your abdominals. Inhaling, raise both legs off the floor, extending them out from the hips at the same time. Hold for a few moments, then breathe out as you lower the legs again. Relax. Repeat four or five times (increasing to ten over time). End with a few Knee Bends.

HELPFUL HINT
Don't try to do the Alternate Lifts unless you can do the other exercises easily. Ideally, practice the Double Leg Lift daily for several weeks before progressing to these.

Alternate Lifts Lie down with your arms by your sides. Slowly raise both legs off the mat, as described above. Hold, then lower them back down to the mat and relax. Turn your head so that you are face-down. Now lift the shoulders, keeping your arms by your side, palms facing up. Again, hold, then release and relax. Repeat the Alternate Lifts four or five times, then do a few Knee Bends.

HELPFUL HINT
Keep a sense of relaxation in the neck and face—particularly the jaw—and do not push the head back as you lift up. If you experience any discomfort in the back while doing these exercises, stop immediately and do some Knee Bends.

Abdominal Curl and Oblique Lift

These exercises serve to strengthen the abdominal muscles, which help to support the back. Work slowly and smoothly, keeping the neck and face muscles relaxed. You should not experience any pain when doing the curls; if you do, your technique may be incorrect and you may need to seek advice from a physiotherapist or qualified fitness trainer. Keep breathing steadily throughout—do not hold your breath—and be sure to keep the face and neck relaxed as you lift up.

1 Start with your feet flat on the floor, knees together. Bring your hands over the head and rest them, palms up, on the floor (if this feels uncomfortable, keep them by your sides, palms down). Contract your abdominals. Exhaling, raise the knees up toward the chest. Do not let your back arch up: keep your tailbone tucked in so that the back flattens slightly against the floor.

2 Continuing to contract your abdominals, raise your sitting bones to bring the knees closer to the chest. Hold for a few moments, then return to the position at the end of step 1. Repeat this several times, moving slowly and breathing normally.

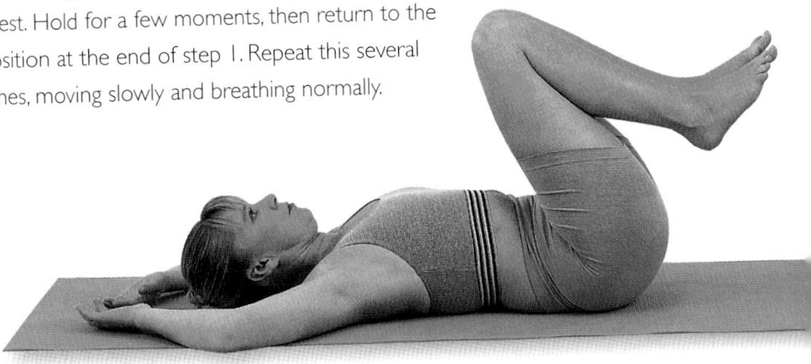

3 As your fitness and strength improve, you can increase the number of curls that you do. You can also increase the stretch by bringing your knees farther into your chest, as shown here. It is helpful to point the feet slightly as you do this.

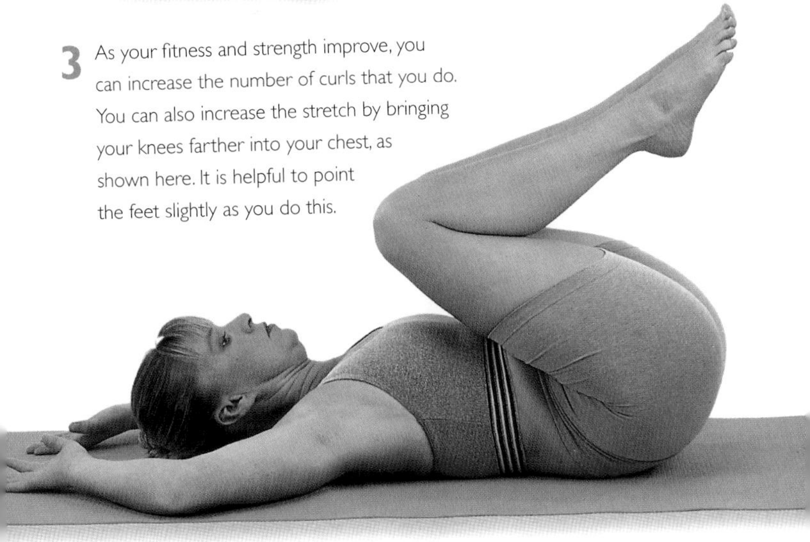

Oblique Shoulder Lift

❶ Lie on your back and bend your knees, placing the feet flat on the mat. Draw your sitting bones forward and upward to flatten the lower back slightly. Bend your left arm, placing your fingers behind the left ear. Extend the right arm out to the side. Contract your abdominals and inhale.

❷ Exhaling, lift up your left shoulder as far as feels comfortable (do not force this movement). You should feel a slight stretch down your side. Keep the face and neck relaxed, letting them follow the movement of your shoulder. Now inhaling, lower yourself back to the ground. Repeat four or five times, then do the same on the other side.

Stretch and Relax

After doing strengthening exercises, it is essential that you release any accumulated tension in the back with some gentle forward bends and stretches. Breathe deeply as you do these exercises, to help create a feeling of relaxation and ease in the body. Then lie down in the Relaxation position (*see page 37*) and relax for at least five minutes. You may like to cover yourself with a light blanket at this point.

Forward Bend

Stand tall, feet hip-distance apart and knees bent. Tuck in your tailbone and chin. Drop the head forward, then slowly bend forward, starting from the base of the neck and working down the spine. Let your arms hang down and breathe deeply. To come up, place your hands on your thighs and unfold from the base of the spine, bringing the head up last.

Squat

Stand with your feet wide apart and pointing outward. Contract your abdominals and squat down. Make sure that your knees are in line with your feet and do not extend farther than your toes. Put your hands flat on the floor or rest them on a support. Hold and breathe. To come up, straighten the legs, keeping your spine erect.

HELPFUL HINT

Many people cannot squat down this far. If you find squatting hard, place a chair in front of you and rest your hands on the seat instead of the floor.

Seated Forward Bend

This soothing posture is a good way to lead into the relaxation.

Sit down with your knees bent and your feet flat on the floor. Bend forward and rest your head between your knees. Let your arms extend down the legs and rest your hands on the feet. Relax your shoulders, neck, and face muscles and breathe deeply for a few moments.

General Back Pain

Back pain is very common—almost everyone suffers from it at some point in their lives, and it is the one of the most common reasons for taking time off work. In most cases the pain is short-lived, but the problem can often recur.

It is not always possible to determine the exact reason why a back problem develops, but the site of the pain and how long it lasts can help to pinpoint the likely cause. Many back problems can be treated at home, but persistent, recurrent, or severe pain should be investigated by a doctor. If you suffer from recurrent pain, it may be a sign you need to pay greater attention to protecting your back, as described earlier in this chapter.

Lower back pain

Six out of ten people experience lower back pain every year. The lower back takes most of the

Sites of back pain

Most back pain gets better on its own, but sometimes there is a specific cause that requires medical attention.

❶ Whiplash Pain in the neck may follow a car accident.

❷ Osteoarthritis Wear and tear of the joints can cause pain in the neck, back, or shoulders.

body's weight, and its muscles and ligaments are therefore particularly susceptible to damage.

Pain that comes on suddenly is likely to be muscle strain, caused by strenuous or unfamiliar physical activity. Sometimes a muscle can go into spasm to prevent further damage. If this is the case, certain points on the muscle may feel very painful and your movement will be restricted.

A dull ache that develops gradually is often due to poor postural habits. Pregnant women often suffer from lower back pain, as the weight of the growing baby affects the way they stand and move. Overweight people may also experience problems.

Back pain may also be caused by a prolapse in one of the disks between the vertebrae (known as a "slipped disk," see *page 48*) or there may be pressure on the sciatic nerve (sciatica, see *page 49*). Occasionally the cause may be a disorder in the joints, such as osteoarthritis, or there may be a problem such as a kidney infection.

Many women suffer from cramplike pain in the lower back during their periods. Pain caused by other disorders can also get worse at this time.

❸ **Fibrositis** Inflammation and tenderness in the large muscles of the back may be due to fibrositis.

❹ **Lower back** Aging, posture problems, or general weakness can cause recurrent pain here.

❺ **Sciatica** Pain in the buttock that travels down the leg may be sciatica.

❻ **Bruised coccyx** A fall can cause painful bruising that is slow to heal.

Acute Back Pain

Back problems are categorized as acute or chronic. Acute pain usually comes on suddenly, and it can be so severe that you may not be able to move or straighten up for a while. It usually settles within a few days or weeks. Chronic problems develop gradually and last for 12 weeks or more. An acute problem may become chronic if it is not treated correctly, or if the underlying cause is not resolved; and a chronic problem may lead to an acute attack.

Slipped disk

When an intervertebral disk prolapses, the jelly-like substance inside squeezes out and can press on a nerve.

1 Prolapsed disk

2 Nerve

3 Spinal cord

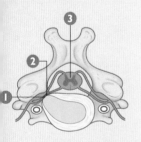

Prolapsed (slipped) disk

The disks that act as shock absorbers between the vertebrae may become worn with age. A sudden movement can cause the jelly-like substance inside the disk to press against the outer edge. If it ruptures, the disk material can squeeze through—this is known as a prolapse. The disk and surrounding tissues may then press on a nerve root or the spinal cord, causing severe pain. If the spinal cord is affected, there may be weakness in the leg or other parts of the body, and urgent medical attention is required.

Pain caused by a slipped disk usually comes on suddenly, but can sometimes develop gradually over a period of time. It generally subsides after several weeks, although the disk is permanently damaged. Pain-killers and physiotherapy are the usual treatment, but sometimes an anti-inflammatory may be injected close to the nerve. Occasionally surgery is needed. Chiropractic and osteopathy can help.

Sciatica

Sciatica is a sharp pain that can be felt anywhere in the area supplied by the sciatic nerves (shown in blue below, running from the spinal cord). Often the pain starts on one side of the back (which goes into spasm) and then runs down the buttock and leg.

Sciatica is the result of pressure on the sciatic nerve. This may be due to a prolapsed disk, to swelling around an injured muscle or to poor posture. Pain-killers help to relieve the pain. Other useful treatments are physiotherapy, osteopathy, chiropractic, and acupuncture.

Injuries

Car headrests

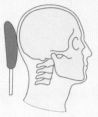

To protect yourself from whiplash when traveling in a car, make sure that the headrest is properly adjusted. It should support the back of your head when you lean back.

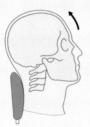

If the headrest reaches only as far as the top of the neck, it provides no support and can be positively harmful, exacerbating the effect of a collision from behind.

Whiplash

Whiplash injuries usually occur when a car has braked very suddenly or if it is hit from behind. The impact causes the head to jerk violently forward and then backward. This sudden jerking can cause damage to the vertebrae, as well as affecting the soft tissues and nerves of the neck.

Symptoms may occur immediately or they may take a day or two to appear. They include pain and stiffness, headache and weakness, and tingling in the shoulders and arms. Some people experience problems for several months. Pain-killers and ice packs can help to relieve the pain, and your doctor may recommend wearing a surgical collar (*see right*). Physiotherapy, chiropractic, osteopathy, and acupuncture can all be beneficial.

Facet joint injuries

The facet joints connect the vertebrae to each other. They help to give the spine stability, but they can easily be damaged by a sudden twisting movement or by a condition such as osteoarthritis. The damaged joint can become inflamed, and it may then press on the surrounding tissues, causing pain in the affected area and sometimes in the buttocks too. Pain-relieving medication, together with treatment from a specialist such as a physiotherapist, osteopath, or chiropractor, is the most common recommendation.

Fractured or slipped vertebra

A vertebra can fracture as a result of a bad fall, a traffic accident, or a heavy blow. In some cases, a fractured vertebrae can cause damage to the spinal cord, which may lead to paralysis or even death. If a fracture is suspected, it is essential that the person remains still while someone contacts the emergency services. Surgery may be needed.

A minor fracture, such as a crack in one of the bony protuberances from each vertebra, can be very painful, but does not cause any permanent damage. Given time, the fracture will heal by itself, and the only treatment is pain relief.

Occasionally one vertebra can slip forward (a condition known as spondylolisthesis). This can occur after a fracture caused by over-stretching or as the result of osteoarthritis or injury. Treatment may involve wearing a brace or having physiotherapy to strengthen the muscles around the vertebra.

Bruised coccyx

A fall on the coccyx can cause bruising or a fracture, which could take months to heal. Osteopathy or chiropractic can be of benefit, and you may find it helps to sit on an air cushion.

A bad fall can cause bruising or a fracture, which may be very painful and take months to heal.

Surgical neck collar

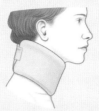

If you are suffering from whiplash, a doctor may recommend that you wear a surgical collar. This provides support for the head and neck, and prevents you from making any jarring movements that could slow down the healing process.

Posture Problems

When looked at from behind, a normal spine looks straight. If observed from the side, however, it curves gently in, out, and in again, making a shallow S-shape. Some people develop an abnormal curvature of the spine, usually as a result of poor posture. This can lead to chronic pain, and it can also increase the risk of a prolapsed disk and other problems.

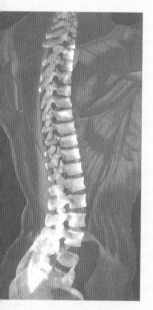

In lordosis, the lumbar spine curves in too much, creating an excessively hollow back.

Lordosis and kyphosis

People with lordosis have an excessive inward curve in the small of their back (the lumbar region). They stand in a slouched position, with the stomach pushed forward and the buttocks sticking out. Lordosis frequently affects people who are overweight, because they tend to lean backward to compensate for the excess weight they carry at the front. It can also affect women who are in the later stages of pregnancy.

People with kyphosis have an exaggerated outward curve in the top of the back (the thoracic spine), creating a hump. They sometimes also develop lordosis, since the lumbar spine curves inward to compensate. Kyphosis can develop in childhood, for no obvious reason. Osteoarthritis and osteoporosis are other possible causes, as well as poor postural habits.

If you think you may have kyphosis or lordosis, you should see your doctor, who can give you advice on how to improve your posture. A physiotherapist may recommend exercises to strengthen the muscles supporting the spine.

The Alexander technique can be a good way of retraining the body to stand and sit correctly. Osteopathy and chiropractic can also help.

Scoliosis

In scoliosis, the spine twists abnormally to the right or to the left. The person may walk abnormally and suffer from recurrent back pain. Scoliosis usually affects children or adolescents. It may be present at birth, or it may develop if, say, one leg is shorter than the other.

Scoliosis needs to be carefully monitored. Wherever possible, the underlying cause is addressed—if the legs are of unequal length, for example, orthopedic shoes may be needed. A back brace may be worn if the problem seems to be progressing. Very occasionally, surgery is recommended for this condition.

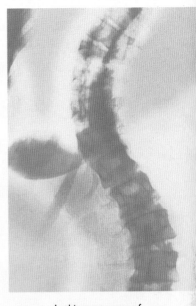

In this severe case of scoliosis, the spine is twisting to one side, so that it forms an S-shape.

Kyphosis

Kyphosis often worsens if left untreated. It is important to seek specialized advice if you think you have abnormal curvature of the spine.

❶ **Normal curvature of the spine** Here the spine curves gently inward at the lumbar region, and out again at the top of the back.

❷ **Spine with kyphosis** Here the exaggerated curve at the top of the back forces the neck forward, creating a "hunchback."

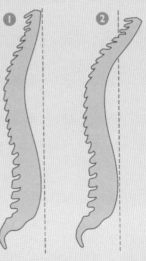

Disorders of the Spine

Our spine is subject to disease and wear and tear, like any other part of the body. The vertebrae become less dense and more vulnerable to fracture with age. The intervertebral discs become thinner and the joints may be affected by osteoarthritis. Other diseases such as osteoporosis can also affect the spine.

Wear and tear

This colored X-ray shows damage to a spine affected by osteoarthritis—you can see the bone spurs sticking out from the vertebrae.

❶ Facet joint

❷ Vertebra

❸ Osteophytes and narrowed cartilage disk

❹ Normal cartilage disk

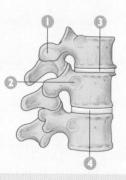

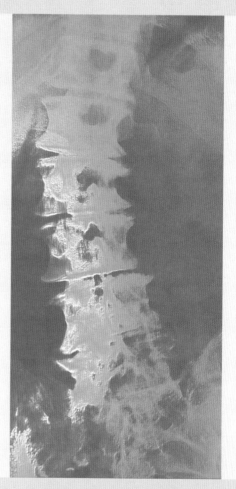

Osteoarthritis (spondylosis)

Osteoarthritis is degeneration of the joints as a result of wear and tear. It is very common: most people over the age of 60 are affected to some extent, although not everyone develops symptoms. The condition usually affects weight-bearing joints such as the hips and knees (see pages 112–13). When osteoarthritis affects the spine, it is called spondylosis. It is most common in the lower back (lumbar spondylosis) and the neck (cervical spondylosis).

Spondylosis causes the protective cartilage in the vertebrae to become eroded. Bone spurs, called osteophytes, can form and may restrict movement, although often they cause no symptoms. The joints can become inflamed, and they and the osteophytes may press on one of the spinal nerves, causing severe pain.

The condition is not reversible, but it will not necessarily get worse. The symptoms can be relieved with pain-killers, anti-inflammatory medication, and heat treatment. Your doctor may also recommend special exercises to maintain movement in the spine. Very occasionally, surgery is recommended—usually if there is damage to a nerve.

Osteoarthritis can be prevented by taking regular moderate exercise and by losing excess weight. These measures can also help to control symptoms.

Ankylosing spondylitis

This inflammatory disease starts in the pelvic joints and spreads up the back.

Ankylosing spondylitis usually affects young men. Early symptoms include lower back pain and stiffness. There is an increasing loss of mobility in the spine, and pain in the upper back. Attacks vary in severity and may last a few weeks. In severe cases the bones may fuse together, and this can lead to the stooped posture shown below.

There is no cure, but the disease may stop its progression at any point. Anti-inflammatories and pain-killers relieve symptoms, and exercises can help to maintain mobility.

Other disorders

Right: Inside our bones is a honeycomb of spongy bone. Osteoporotic bone, shown here, is less dense than normal, so it lacks strength and stability and is more prone to fractures.

Below: Back pain can strike at any age, but is more likely to occur in the elderly, whose bones are already weakened by wear and tear and increasing brittleness.

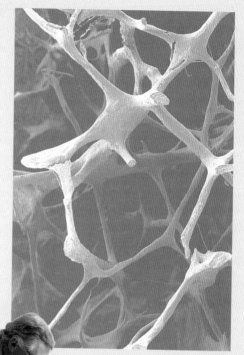

Osteoporosis

As we grow older, our bones become thinner and less dense. In severe cases, the bones become brittle and more liable to break —this is the widespread condition that is known as osteoporosis.

People with osteoporosis may suffer a fracture after a relatively minor fall or, occasionally, even after a violent cough or sudden awkward movement. The vertebrae can become squashed and misshapen; a spinal nerve may then become trapped, causing severe pain. Another effect is that the outward curve of the upper back can become exaggerated (kyphosis, see *page 52*), and this can lead to chronic back pain and loss of mobility.

Anyone can develop osteoporosis, but it is most likely to affect post-menopausal women, and can occur after long-term treatment with corticosteroids. People who are very thin are also at greater risk of developing the condition.

Eating a healthy diet that is rich in calcium and vitamin D (see *pages 88–9*) will help both to prevent osteoporosis and to stop the condition getting worse. Regular weight-bearing exercise is also recommended (under the advice of your doctor) to help improve bone density. Biphosphonate drugs may be prescribed to reduce the risk of fractures. Menopausal women should discuss the subject with their doctor, and might be advised to take HRT (hormone replacement therapy) to reduce the risk of osteoporosis in later life.

Paget's disease

Our bones are constantly being broken down and renewed. In Paget's disease, the rate of new growth accelerates, causing affected bones to become excessively large and deformed (see *page 95*). Paget's disease can affect any area of the body, but the vertebrae are commonly affected. Often there are no symptoms, although some people experience persistent bone pain, which may manifest as a dull ache or a sharp shooting pain in the lower back, which then radiates down the buttocks and legs. Pain-relieving or anti-inflammatory drugs are used to control symptoms, and other medication (biphosphonate drugs) may be given in order to slow the progression of the disease.

Cancer

The spine can be affected by cancer, although this is a very rare cause of back pain.

Tumors can develop in the spine, but more often spread here from elsewhere (secondary cancer). They can affect the bones of the spine, the soft tissues, the nerves, or the lining of the spinal cord. It is worth seeing your doctor for investigative tests if back pain is worse at night or when you lie down; if you are over 50 and suffering from unexplained back pain; or if you have previously been diagnosed with cancer.

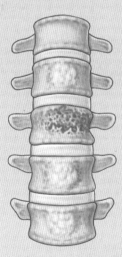

Assessing the Problem

Back pain can often be treated at home. However, you should seek medical advice if you develop immobilizing back pain that does not improve within a day, if you have recurrent attacks, if a chronic condition gets worse, or if you experience other symptoms.

Seeking help

❶ **Call the emergency services** if you have an accident or fall and suspect that you may have hurt your back or your neck. Do not move until help arrives.

❷ **Go to Accident and Emergency** if you are involved in a traffic accident in which your car is hit from behind.

❸ **Ring your family doctor** if disabling back pain develops suddenly and does not improve after a day's rest.

❹ **Call your family doctor** if you have constant back pain which has not improved within 48 hours of self-treatment.

❺ **Call your doctor** if back pain persists or a chronic pain worsens; if you also develop other symptoms; or if you suspect osteoporosis.

❻ **See your doctor immediately** if you have pain or numbness in an arm or leg, loss of bladder or bowel function, or chest pain.

What your doctor may do

Your doctor will ask you to describe your symptoms in detail: for example, the site of the pain; how long it has lasted; whether you had a fall or had been doing strenuous physical activity before the pain started; whether anything makes the pain better or worse; and how your general health is.

Your doctor may then give you a physical examination in which he or she

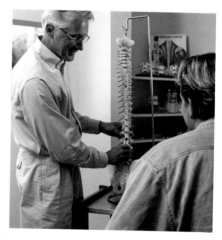

A doctor may be able to help you understand the cause of your pain and how best to manage it.

A physiotherapist may manipulate your joints to ease stiffness and improve mobility. He or she will also teach you to perform specialized exercises, and may also advise you on protecting your back from harm.

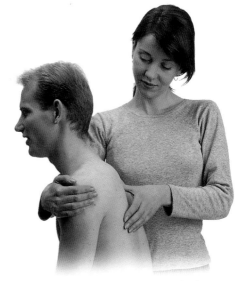

Wearing a corset

Your doctor may recommend that you wear a corset as a short-term measure.

This helps the muscles to relax, and prevents you from making any movements that may exacerbate the problem.

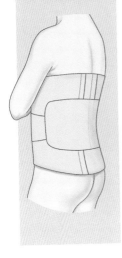

feels your back for tender areas, checks your reflexes, and performs stretches to test your range of movement and your muscle strength.

Often no definite cause is diagnosed, so treatment will focus on relieving symptoms. You may be prescribed pain-killers, anti-inflammatories, muscle-relaxants, or other drugs. Occasionally a corticosteroid may be injected into a painful area.

You may also be given advice on how to improve your posture or the flexibility of your back. If necessary, your doctor will refer you to a physiotherapist, who can recommend specialized exercises or may arrange further tests.

Further investigation

Various tests are done to diagnose the cause of back pain. These include blood tests and X-rays to look for signs of disorders such as Paget's disease or osteoarthritis; and CT or MRI scans if there is evidence of a prolapsed disk. If osteoporosis is suspected, you will be offered a bone-density test, which uses low-dose X-rays.

Simple Self-Treatment

Bed rest used to be the standard advice for bad backs, but most specialists now recommend that you continue with a normal life as far as you are able. Acute, disabling pain may make rest necessary, but you should not stay in bed for more than a day or two. Here are some good ways to manage back pain at home.

When pain strikes

The first thing to do when back pain strikes is to try to reduce any pressure on your spine. If possible, lie down on a bed. If you are not at home, lie on the floor.

Find a comfortable position: try lying flat on your back with your knees bent and supported by cushions, and your head and neck resting on another cushion. Or lie on your side with a cushion between bent knees, as shown below. Cover yourself with a light blanket to keep warm.

Try to relax as much as you can. It will help if you take slow, deep breaths. Try to let go of tension with each exhalation—as if you are breathing it

When pain strikes, rest to reduce any strain on your back. Experiment to find a comfortable position that suits you.

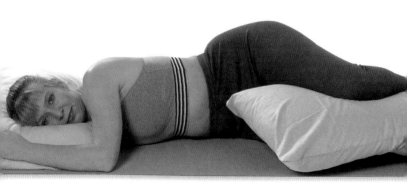

out. Try to change position every so often, to prevent your back from stiffening, and get up every hour or so and walk around.

Relieving pain

Over-the-counter drugs such as non-steroidal anti-inflammatories (ibuprofen) are usually recommended to relieve back pain, but check the precautions given on the pack. Paracetamol is a good all-purpose pain-killer. If these medications do not help, ask your doctor for a stronger one.

Applying heat or cold to the affected area can also be a effective way of relieving pain. Heat is good for muscular aches, while a cold compress or ice pack can reduce inflammation. Try placing an ice pack (or a bag of frozen peas wrapped in a towel) on the area for one minute, then apply a hot towel or covered hot-water bottle for another minute. Repeat, then apply the ice pack again. Do this several times a day.

Regaining mobility

When your pain subsides, it can help to stretch out the back. If possible, continue with your normal activities, but avoid lifting or straining. Try the exercises on the following page, but ask your doctor if you are unsure of their suitability for you.

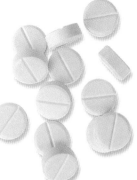

Pain-relieving anti-inflammatories, such as ibuprofen, are available from any pharmacist.

A hot towel applied to the back may help to relieve muscular aches and pains.

Stretching out the Lower Back

These exercises provide a gentle stretch for the back, which can help to relieve pain and improve mobility. You can do them once an hour or so. Work slowly and gently, breathing evenly all the time. Go only as far as feels comfortable. Do the Roll to the Side (*see pages 32–3*) after the Knee Bend, but leave it out if it causes discomfort. As your back starts to improve, you can try the exercises on the following pages.

Knee Bend

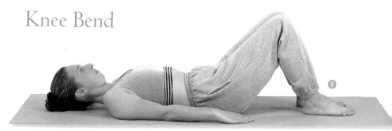

Lie flat on your back with your arms by your sides, Bend the knees so that you can place your feet flat on the floor. Tuck in your chin. Contract your abdominal muscles and tuck in your tailbone, tilting your sitting bones forward and upward slightly, so that the small of your back flattens toward the floor. Take several slow deep breaths, and relax.

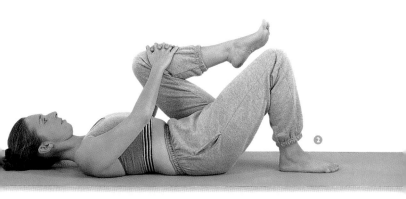

2 Very slowly raise the left leg. Bring your hands around your shin—or, if it feels easier, around the upper thigh, just below the knee. Gently pull your leg closer toward your chest, stopping if you feel any discomfort. Hold this position for a few moments, then return to the floor. Repeat with the right leg.

3 Now raise both knees, again working very slowly. Clasp your hands around your shins (or around the upper thighs) and pull your legs as close to your chest as possible without causing any discomfort. Hold for a few moments and breathe evenly. Then release. Repeat steps 2 and 3 two more times.

HELPFUL HINT

Rest your head on a cushion or a couple of books if this feels more comfortable. You can do the Knee Bend in bed, to prepare your muscles for getting up.

Encouraging Mobility

These flexibility exercises are useful once you have regained some of your mobility. Do them only if you can do the previous exercises easily and without discomfort. Do not try to do them all when you first start—begin with the Pelvic Tilt and Forward Bend, and add the Spinal Twist and Side Stretch (*see pages 66–7*) when your condition improves. You can do them several times a day.

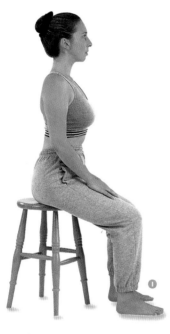

2 Now bring your sitting bones forward and upward, so that your tailbone is tucked in. Hold for a few moments, breathing normally. This is the position you want to adopt in all the exercises. Repeat three or four times, ending with your sitting bones forward and tailbone tucked in.

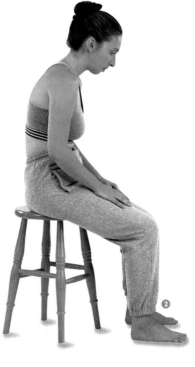

Pelvic Tilt

Sit up straight on a chair or stool, with your feet hip-distance apart and flat on the floor. Roll your sitting bones backward, so that you exaggerate the arch in your back. Do not go too far —this action should be painless.

Forward Bend

1 Sit toward the front of a chair or stool. Your feet should be hip-distance apart and flat on the floor, hands resting gently on your thighs. Keep your tailbone and chin tucked in. Relax your shoulders. Contract your abdominal muscles.

> **HELPFUL HINT**
>
> Be very aware of the limitations of your back when doing this exercise. You may find that you need only bend the head and neck forward in order to feel a stretch.

2 Slowly drop your head toward your chest, then very gently bend forward. Start from the base of the neck and work all the way down the spine, vertebra by vertebra. Slide your hands to your knee as you bend forward. Hold this position for a few moments, breathing normally. Then slowly unfold, from the base of the spine upward. Bring the head up last.

Spinal Twist and Side Stretch

These exercises should be done after the Pelvic Tilt and Forward Bend (*see pages 64–5*). As the flexibility of your spine improves, you can increase the number of repetitions from one to five. Take care not to force the twist, and tighten your abdominal muscles to give support to the spine.

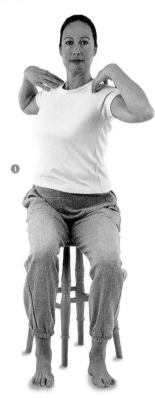

2 Twist slightly more, but only as far as feels comfortable. Then return to the center and repeat on the other side. Keep your head in an erect central position at all times, and do not let the shoulders tense.

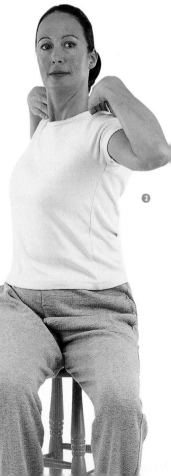

Sit tall, bringing your sitting bones forward and upward so that you can tuck in the tailbone. Place your fingertips on your shoulders, as shown. Contract your abdominals. Breathing in, very slowly bring your left shoulder forward and your right shoulder back, to twist the spine. You should feel a slight stretch along the right side. Keep the hips stable. Hold, breathing normally.

2 Breathe in and come up to your original sitting position. Then breathe out and bend slowly to the right in the same way. Tighten the abdominal muscles and keep your hips stable throughout.

1 Sit upright, with your feet hip-distance apart and flat on the floor and your arms by your sides. Check that your tailbone is tucked in, and contract the abdominal muscles. Breathing out, slowly bend to the left. Keep your hips centered and your head in line with the spine as you bend.

HELPFUL HINT

You need a stool or a chair without arms to do the Side Stretch. Start the bend from the shoulder, letting the movement travel down the spine toward the lower back.

Relieving Shoulder and Neck Pain

These exercises work to improve mobility in the shoulders and neck. They are a good way of releasing tension and can be done several times during the day. Build your flexibility bit by bit, gradually increasing the number of repetitions from one to four. Work very slowly and do not force the neck too far. If you feel any pain, stop. Check the suitability of the exercises with your doctor if you have a chronic condition, such as osteoarthritis (*see page 55*).

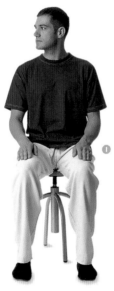

2 Keeping your head erect, turn back to the center and then turn to the left in one slow, continuous movement. Hold for a few moments, breathing normally, and then turn to the center. Repeat up to four times.

Head Turn

Sit upright. Bring your sitting bones forward and upward, so that your tailbone is tucked in. Rest your hands on your thighs. Very slowly turn your head to the right as far as is comfortable. Hold for a few moments, breathing evenly.

3 Now drop the head forward very slowly, so that you bring your chin to your chest—or as close as it will comfortably go. Keep your back straight and do not let your shoulders tense.

4 Slowly lift the head up and then back, pointing the chin upward. Be sure that you do not drop the head back quickly or force the neck farther than it will comfortably go. Then slowly return it to the upright position. Keep breathing evenly throughout the exercise.

Sideways Tilt

When moving the neck, it is important that you do not make any sudden movements. All the tilts should be slow and smooth. As your flexibility improves, increase the number of repetitions from one to four.

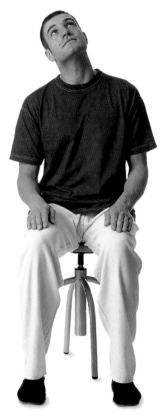

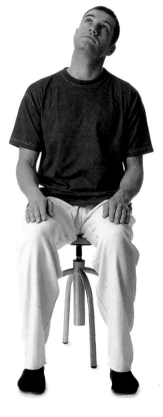

1 Sit upright with your feet flat on the floor and your hands on your upper thighs. Slowly tilt your head to the right, lifting your chin so that you face upward. You should feel a gentle stretch on the left side, from the jaw and down the neck.

2 Return your head to its central position, and then slowly tilt it to the left. Feel the stretch on the right side of your face and neck. Keep your shoulders level and relaxed as you move the head. Keep breathing steadily throughout the exercise.

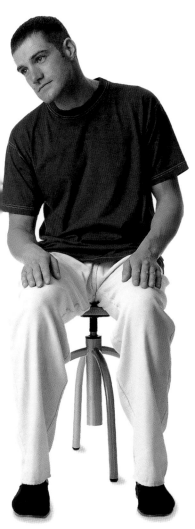

Shoulder Hunch

❶ Relax the shoulders. Now lift your left shoulder up, as close to the ear as it will comfortably go. Release it.

❷ Now raise the right shoulder, and release. Repeat several times. Then lift and release both shoulders at once. Do this several times.

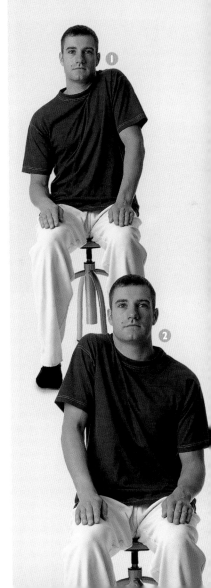

3 Tilt your head to the right side, facing forward. Gently drop the chin, moving it across your chest and then up to the left, as if you were tracing a semicircle in the air with your chin. Repeat the action, this time starting from the left and moving to the right. Return your head to its central position.

Exercises for Sciatica

These exercises are recommended by traditional Chinese doctors as a way of relieving sciatica. Do not do them when the pain is acute; they are intended to speed a recovery that has already started. Go only as far as the Seated Leg Stretch (*see page 74*) at first, then add the other exercises one by one as your condition improves. Do not do the final Toe Touch (*see page 77*) until you can do the others with ease.

Sciatica (*see page 49*) can have several causes (including a prolapsed disk) and it is important that you get a diagnosis from your doctor and check that these exercises are suitable for you.

I Start by gently tapping the lower body —this is a Chinese technique that helps release tension and boost the circulation. You will need a wooden baton wrapped in layers of cloth. Tap the lower back for a few minutes, then work on the hips and thighs. You can do this three or four times a day.

2 Lie on your back, arms by your sides, knees bent and feet flat on the floor. Bring your sitting bones forward and upward so that your tailbone is tucked in. Contract your abdominals, then slowly straighten the left leg as much as you can—do not force it. Hold for a few moments, then release. Repeat the stretch on the right leg.

3 Bring your knees together. Keeping
your abdominals tight, exhale and
very slowly raise the knees toward
your chest. Place the hands in
between the knees. Push your
knees outward with your hands,
while at the same time using your
knees to push the hands together.
Do this for about 30 seconds,
breathing normally, then release the
pressure. Exhaling, lower your legs
and return your feet to the floor.

4 Lie on the side that is unaffected
by sciatica. Rest your head and neck
on a pillow and bend the knees,
resting your upper arm on your hip
and bending the lower arm in a
comfortable position. Slowly swing
the affected leg backward and
forward for about 30 seconds.
Keep your tailbone tucked in
and your abdominals tight.

HELPFUL HINT

During acute attacks of sciatica,
massaging the area may help. Seek
specialist advice from a physiotherapist,
or see an acupuncturist or osteopath.

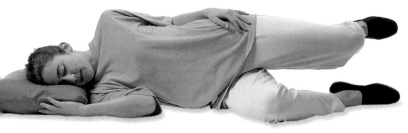

Seated Leg Stretch

1 Sit toward the front of a chair with your feet flat on the ground. Rest your hands on the seat behind you and lean back slightly—this helps to ease any pressure on the lower back. Contract your abdominal muscles. Now slowly raise your left leg and extend it in front of you.

2 Bend the leg, bringing the knee toward your chest as far as feels comfortable. Continue extending and then bending the leg, up to a maximum of eight repetitions. Stop if this feels uncomfortable at any point. Then repeat the exercise on your right leg.

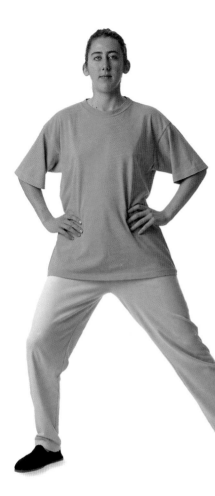

Side to Side

Stand in a wide stance, knees bent and feet pointing out. Tuck in the chin and tailbone. Rest your hands on your hips. Slowly shift your weight onto your right leg, bending this leg a little more and letting the left one straighten. Keep your hips facing forward and your back straight. Now shift back to the center, and to the left. Repeat up to eight times on each side.

Deep Bend

❶ Sit at the front of a chair, with legs bent. Rest your hands on your thighs.

❷ As you exhale, bend down from the waist, sliding the arms down the legs. Go only as far as needed to feel a stretch, and drop the head last. Inhale and come up slowly, lifting the head last. Repeat the process.

Waist and Back Bend

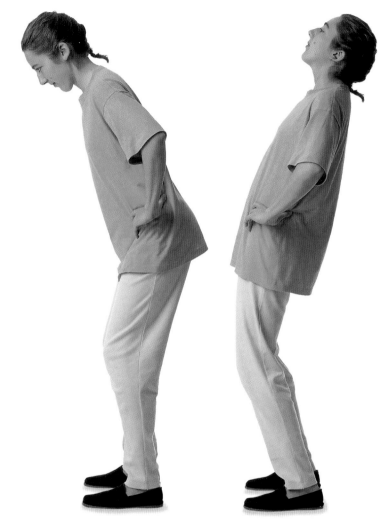

1 Stand tall with your knees bent and your feet shoulder-distance apart. Rest your hands on your hips and contract your abdominals. Bend forward from the waist, keeping the back straight and the head in line with the spine. Do not go too far. Come up slowly.

2 Now bend slightly backward, again bending from the waist and keeping the head in line with the spine. Do not force the movement farther than feels comfortable. You can repeat the bends up to eight times, bending a little farther each time, if you can.

Leg Swing

Stand tall, with your chin and tailbone tucked in. Hold onto the back of a sturdy chair for support. Raise the affected leg, keeping it slightly bent. Slowly swing it backward and forward for a couple of minutes. Stop if you feel tired, or if the swinging feels uncomfortable.

Toe Touch

Sit toward the front of a chair, with your legs extended in front of you and your heels resting on the ground. Breathe out and bend slowly forward, extending the hands toward the toes (do not worry if you cannot reach very far; the important thing is to bend without straining). Breathe in as you come up. Repeat once more.

Exercises for Back Pain in Pregnancy

Most pregnant women experience lower-back pain at some stage or other, particularly during the final months. These exercises gently stretch out the lower back, which can help to alleviate pain. You can do them several times a day. However, do not lie flat on your back after 30 weeks—do only the seated exercises after this point.

2 Gently contract your abdominal muscles. Shift the sitting bones backward, so that you create a slightly deeper arch in your lower back—you should feel a gentle stretch. Return to the correct position, and repeat this gentle rocking several times. Keep breathing evenly as you do the exercise.

Seated Pelvic Tilt

1 Sit on a stool, with both feet placed flat on the floor. Shift your sitting bones forward and upward to bring the pelvis into the correct position.

Supine Pelvic Tilt

1 Lie flat on your back (but not after 30 weeks), bending your knees so that you can place your feet flat on the floor. Your knees should be hip-distance apart. Gently contract your abdominals and tilt your sitting bones forward and upward to bring the lower back as close as possible to the floor (do not force it). Hold and breathe evenly.

HELPFUL HINT

Work very gently, and do not push your body farther than feels natural and comfortable. Stop straight away if you feel any pain. You can rest your head and neck on a cushion if you like.

2 Release the sitting bones and then draw them backward, so that you emphasize the arch in your lower back. Again, do not force this movement. Now, tilt the sitting bones forward slightly, so that your pelvis is in the correct position. Repeat steps 1 and 2 four times. Then relax for a few minutes. To come up, roll onto your side and use your arms to push yourself up.

Complementary Therapies

Complementary therapies such as osteopathy and chiropractic can be very successful in alleviating back pain, and many doctors now recommend them. Ask your doctor if he or she can direct you to a practitioner; otherwise contact the relevant professional association. Tell your practitioner if you have had treatment for back problems, have any other medical condition, or are pregnant. You should also let your doctor know that you intend having treatment.

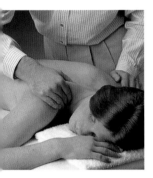

Research has shown that joint manipulation can be an effective way of improving back pain.

Osteopathy

Osteopathy is widely respected by doctors and is often the first choice of therapy for those suffering from musculoskeletal problems. Gentle manipulations, stretches, and sharp thrusts are used to restore the natural alignment of the spine and joints, while the soft tissues are manipulated using massage. Osteopathy can relieve problems caused by poor posture, stress, and injury.

On your first visit, an osteopath will take a full medical history. He or she may also arrange X-rays or other diagnostic tests to check for the underlying causes of your problem. You will usually

Adjusting the spine

Osteopaths and chiropractors use a range of physical adjustments to relieve distortions in the spine. Here, a chiropractor applies pressure using a twisting motion. This helps to realign the vertebrae and restore the spine's flexibility.

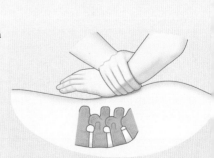

be asked to undress to your underwear and perform some simple movements—such as sitting down or walking. This lets the practitioner assess how you hold yourself and move. You will also need to lie on a special couch, so that the osteopath can examine your spine.

Osteopathic treatment usually takes 15–20 minutes. It should not be painful, but you may feel and hear a "pop" as the bones of a joint slip back into place. You may feel stiff for a day or two afterward. Some people notice a marked improvement after just one session, although several sessions are usually needed.

Chiropractic

Like osteopathy, chiropractic is a method of joint manipulation, but slightly different techniques are used. It emphasizes the idea that the spine is central to good health; misalignments here can cause pain and immobility and may have an effect on other areas of the body. Chiropractors use precisely applied pressure, massage, and vertebral manipulation to bring the spine back into proper alignment. McTimoney chiropractors use a special technique, which is very gentle, and tend to work on the whole body in each session.

Like osteopaths, chiropractors take a full medical history. They may carry out x-rays and other diagnostic tests, as well as examining your body and asking you to perform simple movements in order to assess the problem.

Regular chiropractic or osteopathic treatment can help a pregnant woman adjust to changes in her posture and may help to prevent back strain.

Safety

Osteopathy and chiropractic are considered very safe therapies. However, they are not suitable for people with a severe prolapsed disk, a recent fracture, advanced osteoporosis, or other bone disorders. If you have a serious health problem, always discuss the benefits of complementary treatment with your doctor.

Other Helpful Therapies

Some people find massage very helpful for certain back problems. The Alexander technique, yoga, and shiatsu can also be beneficial, particularly as ways of preventing back problems from recurring. Ask your doctor for advice if you are not sure which therapy is most suitable for you.

The Alexander technique

The aim of the Alexander technique is to train people to maintain good posture at all times. It is based on the idea that most of us have become accustomed to holding ourselves in ways that are unnatural. It can be an excellent therapy for preventing general back pain and may help to alleviate problems associated with poor posture.

In the Alexander technique, you practice simple actions such as getting up from a chair without hunching or twisting your body.

The Alexander technique shows you how to sit, stand, and move so that you place minimum strain on the muscles and joints. Simple actions are practiced to help train the body into what are known as new "patterns of use." Eventually better posture should become automatic. The teaching is usually given on a one-to-one basis, and you will also be given simple exercises (such as answering the phone in a certain way) to practice in between sessions. Most people need 20–30 lessons, with regular follow-ups.

Yoga therapy

Yoga is a system of physical postures that can be used to improve your alignment, strength, and flexibility. Regular practice can help to prevent back problems, and specific postures can be used to alleviate pain. Yoga is also often recommended by doctors as a relaxation technique. However, some postures may exacerbate a back problem, especially if done incorrectly, so if you suffer from back pain,

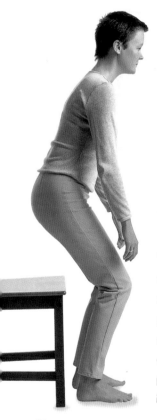

it is important that you seek out a remedial class with an experienced, qualified teacher, and that you discuss your medical history with him or her. Choose a small class where you will receive one-to-one attention.

Massage

A professional massage can be helpful for some muscular problems. Most masseurs use Swedish techniques, which include stroking, kneading, and pummeling, to manipulate the soft tissues. These help to release tension from the muscles and increase the circulation of blood and nutrients.

A major benefit of massage is its relaxing effect, and it may be particularly helpful to people whose problem is associated with stress. Sports masseurs use the same techniques, but they often take a more vigorous approach and are trained to deal with muscular injuries.

Shiatsu

Shiatsu is a Japanese form of massage. Like acupuncture, it is based on the idea that healing energy flows through the body. Finger pressure and gentle stretches are used to release any blockages and stimulate energy flow. Shiatsu is best used as a preventative therapy, although it can also be employed to soothe simple back pain. However, this treatment is not suitable if you suffer from osteoporosis or if you are pregnant.

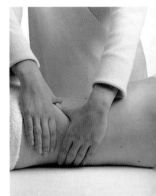

Massage helps to release tension from the muscles, and it can feel highly relaxing.

Shiatsu practitioners may use their hands, elbows, knees, and feet during treatment.

Further Techniques

Acupuncture has had success in treating lower back pain and sciatica, and many people find that the relaxing effects of reflexology can help soothe simple back pain. Aromatherapy oil or homeopathic remedies can also be used to promote healing.

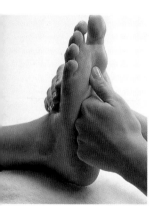

Reflexology can have a relaxing effect on the whole body, including the back and shoulders.

Lavender oil is good for stress, and can help to soothe muscular aches and pains.

Acupuncture

In traditional acupuncture, fine needles are inserted in certain points of the body to redirect the flow of the body's energy and thus stimulate healing. It is often recommended for sciatica and pain relief. US studies have shown that acupuncture can help relieve neck and lower back pain; it may also ease osteoarthritis. You may feel a "tug" when the needles are inserted. Some relief may be felt on the first session, but several treatments are usually needed.

Reflexology

In reflexology, pressure is applied to the feet in order to promote healing elsewhere in the body. Like traditional acupuncture, this technique is based on the idea that good health depends on the free flow of energy around the body. Many people find it relaxing, and it can help to relieve back problems connected to poor posture or stress.

Natural help

Essential oils that may be helpful for muscular problems include lavender, ginger, and marjoram. Dilute well in a base oil and rub into the back, or add a few drops to the bath. Homeopathic remedies, such as arnica or rhus tox, may also help —seek advice from a qualified practitioner.

Your Bones

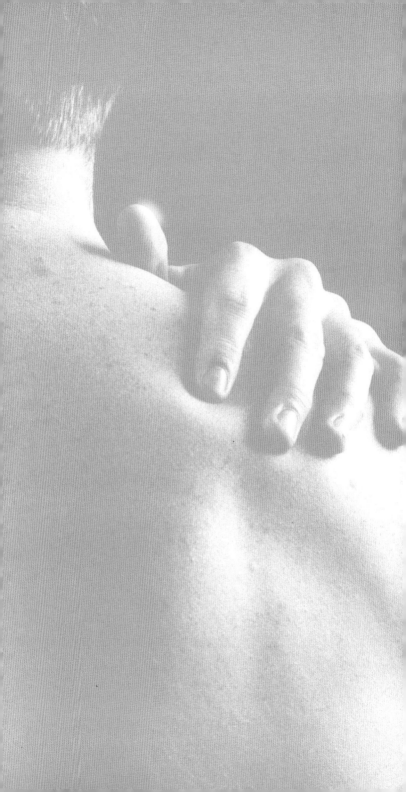

Healthy Bones

Bones are made up of collagen (protein) and minerals. We tend to think that our bones are inert and unchanging, but in fact they are living tissue supplied by a network of nerves and blood vessels. Bones are constantly being broken down and rebuilt to meet the needs of the body. Your age, the type of exercise that you do, and the foods you eat all have an effect on the strength of your bones.

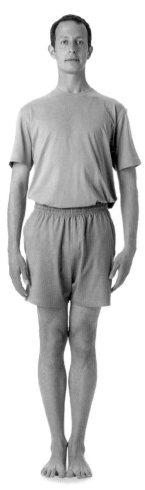

Growing bones

When we are born, our bones consist mostly of cartilage tissue, which is quite soft. Through childhood and early adulthood, the bones grow longer, larger, and harder. Even when we stop growing, our bones continue to increase in density —which is what gives them their strength. They need a constant supply of calcium and other minerals to stay strong.

Bones are at maximum density (peak bone mass) between the ages of 25 and 30. In later life, more calcium tends to leave the bones than is replaced. The bones then become lighter and weaker, and the risk of fractures increases.

Weight-bearing exercise

To help maintain your bones, you need to do weight-bearing exercise on a regular basis. This is any activity that you do on your feet, with your bones supporting your weight.

Standing still or walking puts little strain on your bones. But whenever you take a step, jump, or kick a ball, your bones withstand an impact that can be six times as much as your body weight. They respond to this stress by becoming denser and stronger. Fast walking or jogging are ideal forms of weight-bearing exercise, but any physical activity —including gardening or housework—will help. Other good forms of weight-bearing exercise include aerobics, step, tennis, football, or dance. Weight-training in the gym is a good way of building bone density in the upper body.

Most people should do at least 30 minutes of exercise three or four times a week. You need to increase the amount and intensity of exercise that you do over time in order to sustain its effect on bone density. It is a good idea to check with your doctor before starting any new fitness program, particularly if you have any health problems or if you are over- or underweight.

A fitness program will bring benefits at any age, but ideally you should start young and continue exercising throughout your life. The best time to build your bones' density is when they are still growing, so children and adolescents should be encouraged to exercise on a regular basis. This is extremely important for girls, because women have a higher risk of developing bone problems.

Opposite: Maintaining good posture reduces any unnecessary stress on your bones, and helps to protect your joints.

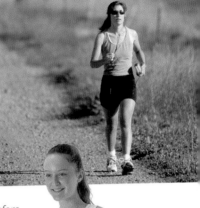

Right and far right: Doing regular weight-bearing exercise from a young age will help build and maintain strong, healthy bones.

Eating for a Strong Frame

To keep your bones healthy and strong, you need to eat a well-balanced diet that is rich in calcium and other minerals, such as magnesium and phosphorus. Spending time outdoors every day, and avoiding smoking and excessive drinking, are other ways that you can help to build strong bones.

Supplements

The best way to meet your calcium needs is through your diet.

Nutritionists suggest that we take in 1000mg of calcium daily—more if you are a pregnant or breastfeeding woman. If you cannot get enough calcium from your diet, talk to a doctor about taking supplements.

Dairy products are the best sources of calcium, but you can also obtain it from other foods.

Essential minerals

Both adults and children should eat calcium-rich foods on a daily basis. The best sources are dairy products such as milk, cheese, and yogurt. You can also get calcium from fish with edible bones, such as anchovies, canned salmon, and sardines. Bread, cereal, pulses, and green leafy vegetables are other good sources of calcium.

Phosphorus works with calcium to lay down new bone tissue. Many calcium-rich foods, such as milk and chicken, also contain phosphorus, so you are unlikely to go short as long as you are meeting your calcium needs. Another mineral that is important is magnesium. It is found in a wide range of foods, including wholegrain cereals, nuts, pulses, and green leafy vegetables. Magnesium deficiency is unlikely, provided you are eating a reasonably balanced diet.

The sunshine vitamin

We need vitamin D in order to absorb calcium properly. This vitamin is manufactured by the body whenever our skin is exposed to sunlight. Any vitamin D that is surplus to our immediate needs can be stored in the liver and accessed during periods when we tend to spend less time outdoors, such as winter.

Taking a short walk outside each day is a good way of ensuring that you are producing enough vitamin D. You can also obtain this nutrient from certain foods, such as oily fish, butter, full-fat milk, some fortified breakfast cereals, and eggs.

What to avoid

Tea, coffee, alcohol, and fizzy drinks hasten the loss of calcium from the body, so they should not be consumed to excess. Wheat bran and salt also have a negative effect, so they should be eaten in moderation.

Smoking increases the loss of bone density, so you should cut down or—better still—give up completely.

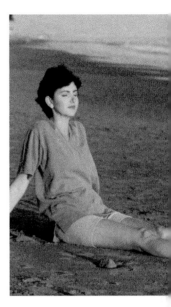

Soaking up the sun stimulates your body into producing vitamin D, which helps you to absorb the calcium you need.

Calcium

Below is the calcium content of some common foods.

Food	Calcium
1 cup milk	290mg
1 cup fortified soya milk	280mg
⅔ cup yogurt	300mg
1¾ oz Cheddar	90mg
2¼ oz tofu	304mg
3 slices bread	100mg
1 egg	90mg
4 oz cabbage	40mg

WHAT CAN GO WRONG

Injuries

The most frequent problem to affect bones is a fracture. This may be the result of an injury—such as a direct blow or a fall—or it may be due to a twisting movement, as may occur during, say, a football game. Any bone can break, but a fracture is most likely to occur in the arms, legs, feet, and hands. Older people commonly break the thighbone or the wrist.

The healing process

Fractures start to heal straight away. A callus forms around the break to protect the bone while healing takes place. This can be seen on an X-ray as early as two weeks after the accident occurs.

❶ Fracture

❷ Callus

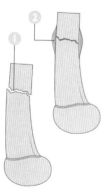

There are two main types of fractures: closed and open. In an open fracture, the broken end of the bone breaks through the skin; in a closed fracture, it remains below the surface.

Fractures are very painful, and the pain increases if you try to move the affected part of the body. The area may be misshapen, swollen, or bruised. An X-ray is usually done to ascertain the exact site of the fracture, and its type.

Types of fracture

Bone fractures are categorized according to the nature of the break.

Transverse fracture This involves a straight break across the width of the bone. It is usually caused by a heavy blow, and often occurs in arms or legs.

Spiral fracture This type of break is caused by a sudden twisting movement. It usually affects the bones of the arm or leg.

Greenstick Here, one side of the bone cracks while the other bends. Greenstick fractures occur only in children, whose bones are more flexible than those of adults.

Comminuted fracture In this type, part of the bone shatters. The pieces may then cause damage to surrounding tissues. A comminuted fracture is caused by a direct blow or impact.

Depressed fracture In this break, an area of bone is dented inward. Depression fractures are most likely to occur in the skull after a blow.

Crush fracture Here the spongy interior of the bone becomes compressed. It usually occurs in the vertebrae of people with osteoporosis.

The main treatment for fractures is to stabilize the bone so that it can heal in the correct position. A plaster or resin cast is commonly used, but sometimes metal rods or screws may be inserted to hold the broken ends together, or an external frame may be pinned to the bone.

Healing takes one to three months, depending on your age and health and the type of fracture. Antibiotics are usually needed if the fracture is open, because it is susceptible to infection.

Broken collarbone

Collarbone fractures generally occur after a fall An arm sling is needed to take the weight off the shoulder joint until the bone ends knit together.

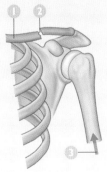

❶ Collarbone

❷ Fracture

❸ Direction of force during a fall

Greenstick fracture

Children's bones are flexible and bendy, so they are less prone to fractures than adult bones.

But if they bend too far, one side of the bone may crack. These fractures can be hard to spot, but they may impede growth: always ask for an X-ray of a suspicious injury.

❶ Greenstick fracture

Comminuted fracture

A comminuted fracture is very painful, and it takes longer to heal than a simple break. It often affects the elbow.

❶ Comminuted fracture

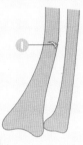

WHAT CAN GO WRONG

Abnormalities

Bones can be pushed out of shape if they become too soft, or if they are constantly put under pressure. Some people are born with an extra rib, which can cause problems if it presses on a nerve.

Site of a bunion

A bunion can be very painful, making walking difficult. If tight shoes continue to rub against the affected area, the skin may be broken and an infection may set in. Antibiotics will then be required.

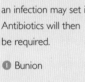

❶ Bunion

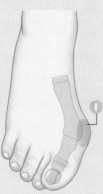

Bunions

In a bunion, the bone at the base of the big toe is deformed and the surrounding tissues are thickened and tender. Bunions usually develop when the foot is regularly squeezed into a tight shoe, which presses on the joint and forces the bone inward.

The underlying cause is a minor bone disorder called hallux valgus. This condition sometimes runs in families. Women are most susceptible to bunions, because they are more likely to wear tight, pointed shoes. Children and young people are particularly vulnerable to developing a bunion, because their bones are still soft. It is therefore essential that they wear correctly fitted shoes.

In its early stages, a bunion should improve if you wear comfortable shoes and a special toe pad—your doctor or a chiropodist can offer advice on this. If the bunion becomes more uncomfortable or pronounced, seek medical advice.

Your doctor may recommend surgery. In this procedure, the protruding part of the bone is removed, and a cut is made lower down so that the remaining bone can be realigned. The area may feel very painful afterward, and it will be six weeks before you can resume normal activities.

Osteomalacia (rickets)

Low levels of calcium and vitamin D can lead to the condition osteomalacia (which is known as rickets when it affects children). It involves a softening of the bones, which become prone to fractures and may be painful. Occasionally the lower legs may develop a curved shape, as they bend under the weight of the body.

The disorder may be caused by an inadequate diet, impaired absorption, or kidney disease. In the developing world, children are rarely affected, but elderly people who are house-bound may be at risk. Treatment involves improving the diet, taking supplements, and treating any underlying condition—such as kidney or intestinal disorders—that might hinder absorption.

Cervical rib syndrome

People with cervical rib syndrome have an extra rib at the base of the neck. Sometimes this can press against the nerves in the neck, causing pain down the inside of one arm. The hand may also be affected: it may feel heavy, weak, cold, or clumsy.

If a cervical rib causes problems, you should see your doctor and ask if you can be referred to a physiotherapist. Special exercises such as shrugging the shoulders can often help to relieve some of the symptoms. In some cases, more serious however, the rib will need to be surgically removed.

What is a cervical rib?

Cervical ribs are hard outgrowths protruding from one of the vertebrae in the neck. They can vary in size from a small bony knob to a complete extra rib. Some people are born with an extra cervical rib, and it is usually harmless. But if it presses against a nerve, it can cause aching and tingling down the arm and in the hand. This is more likely to occur as the person ages and the shoulder starts to sag.

❶ Vertebrae of the neck—the cervical spine

❷ Extra rib

❸ First vertebra of the thoracic (upper spine)

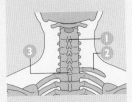

WHAT CAN GO WRONG

Diseases

The most common form of bone disease is osteoporosis, which affects one in four women over the age of 50. Other disorders that affect the bones include Perthes disease and Paget's disease.

Bone density

In people with this bone disease, the strong honeycomb of spongy bone inside affected bones degenerates into a fragile mesh. This can then easily crumble after a fall or injury.

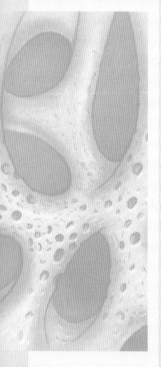

Osteoporosis

Most people experience a loss of bone density and strength as they grow older. In osteoporosis, the process is accelerated and the bones become weak and brittle so that the affected person is vulnerable to fractures, even after a minor fall. The bones that are most likely to be affected are those of the hips, wrists, and spine (see pages 56–7).

Osteoporosis is commonly discovered after a fracture, but there are other warning signs, including unexplained back and hip pain, a reduction in height, and, sometimes, a gradual stooping of the back as the weakened bones of the spine become pressed out of shape. You should see your doctor if you notice any of these symptoms.

Anyone can develop osteoporosis, but women are most at risk, particularly after the menopause when hormonal changes take place. Other risk factors include the use of corticosteroid drugs over a long period, having a low body weight, smoking, and excessive consumption of alcohol.

Osteoporosis is diagnosed by means of a bone-density scan, which uses low-radiation

X-rays. Blood tests and regular X-rays may also be arranged to check for other causes of symptoms. If the diagnosis of osteoporosis is confirmed, hormone replacement therapy might be recommended for some women. Your doctor will also discuss with you ways of increasing your bone strength through diet and regular exercise. Calcium and vitamin D supplements may be prescribed. Sometimes biphosphonates are given to slow bone loss and promote normal bone growth. Osteoporosis cannot be cured, but the progression of the disease can be halted.

Perthes disease

Perthes disease affects children, usually boys, aged between three and ten. It is an abnormality affecting the top of the thigh bone, which temporarily softens and breaks down. The bone is gradually replaced over a period of about 18 months.

Perthes disease causes pain in the hip and knee, and movement may be restricted. The affected leg may become slightly shorter than the other, causing the child to limp.

Seek medical advice if a child develops an unexplained limp or has pain in the knee or hip. Bed rest is needed until any pain subsides; a cast or brace may be used to hold the thighbone in place while the bone re-forms. Affected children will have regular X-rays to monitor the regrowth of the bone. Physiotherapy treatment may also be needed to help improve mobility of the hip as the new bone forms.

Paget's disease

In Paget's disease, areas of bone are broken down and rebuilt at an accelerated rate.

The bones can become soft and deformed (*shown below*), and are also liable to fracture. Any bone can be affected, but the skull, hip, pelvis, spine (*see page 57*), legs, arms, and shoulders are most at risk. When the skull is affected, headaches, blindness, and deafness can occur. Biphosphonate drugs, which promote normal bone growth, are the usual treatment.

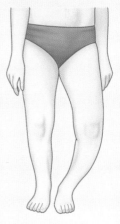

Infections and Tumors

Like any other part of the body, bones are subject to infection. They can also become cancerous. Cancer that starts in the bones is rare, and generally affects children rather than adults. Secondary cancer, in which the disease spreads from another part of the body, is more common in adults.

Benign tumor

Non-cancerous bone tumors are most likely to affect children and young adults. They can occur anywhere, but often develop from the growing cartilage that covers the end of the long bones in the limbs. As the bone lengthens during normal growth, the tumor stays in the original position.

❶ Tumor

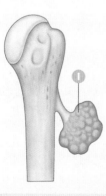

Infections

Bones can become infected—a condition that is known as osteomyelitis. This causes pain and inflammation in the affected area, as well as a sudden increase in body temperature. A nearby joint may also swell up. Osteomyelitis usually affects young children or elderly people, although it can also occur in adults after a fracture.

Osteomyelitis needs to be treated promptly or it may lead to blood poisoning (septicemia). Inflammation inside the bone can also cut off the supply of blood and oxygen, which may affect bone growth or cause the bone tissue to die. The usual treatment is antibiotics, which need to be given intravenously in hospital.

Benign bone tumors

Benign bone tumors are non-cancerous growths that can develop in any part of the bone. They may cause no symptoms, although sometimes they can be painful, especially if they press on a nerve. Occasionally, they can restrict movement, or they may cause the bone to become misshapen. Tumors can also make the bone more liable to fracturing.

Your doctor will arrange an X-ray or MRI (magnetic resonance imaging) scan if a tumor is suspected. Sometimes a small piece of the bone may be removed (a biopsy) and checked for signs of cancer. Non-cancerous bone tumors will normally be surgically removed if they cause problems, grow rapidly or show any signs of becoming cancerous. However, in many cases they may be left in place.

Primary cancer

Cancerous tumors can develop in the bone (primary cancer), but more commonly the disease starts elsewhere in the body and then spreads to the bones (secondary cancer). Primary bone cancer is rare in adults. It is most likely to affect children and young people, usually in the bones of the leg. Symptoms of both types of cancer include pain, tenderness, and swelling in the affected area, as well as an increased vulnerability to fracturing. The pain may increase at night, and when the person stands up or lies down.

Cancer is diagnosed by X-rays, MRI, or CT (computerized tomography) scanning. Other parts of the body, such as the lungs, may also be screened to see if the disease has spread elsewhere. If a diagnosis of primary cancer is confirmed, the tumor will be surgically removed wherever possible. Radiotherapy or chemotherapy is usually performed to destroy any cancer cells left behind. Treatment for primary bone cancer is usually successful, and in most cases the disease does not recur.

Secondaries

Secondary bone tumors are most likely to affect the ribs, pelvis, spine, and skull.

Secondaries (known as metastases) destroy bone tissue, making the bone vulnerable to fracturing (see below). Treatment focuses on the original site, which is often in the lung, kidney, thyroid, or prostate. The bone tumors cannot be surgically removed, but radiotherapy or chemotherapy can help to destroy them.

❶ Secondary tumor

❷ Fracture

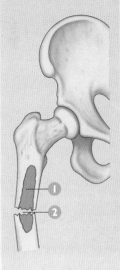

Living with Bone Problems

Bone disorders need medical attention, and they cannot be treated at home. You will usually need to go to hospital for investigative tests to pinpoint the problem. But if you are diagnosed with osteoporosis, there is a lot you can do to help yourself.

Take sensible precautions to help yourself and prevent the risk of fractures and other bone problems.

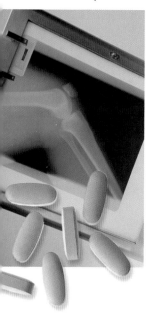

Calcium and vitamin D supplements may be recommended if you suffer from osteoporosis.

When to seek help

You should see your doctor if you experience unexplained bone pain or if you notice swelling or tenderness in the skin over a bone. Loss of height or marked changes in your posture should also be reported to your medical adviser. If a child develops pain in the hip or knee, starts to limp, or has an injury to the arm or leg that looks suspicious, you should seek medical advice as soon as possible.

If you visit your doctor with bone pain, he or she will ask you about your symptoms and will also perform a physical examination. You may be referred to hospital for investigative tests such as X-rays or other scans. If osteoporosis is suspected, a bone-density scan will be done.

If you have one of the risk factors for osteoporosis—if you are a woman approaching the menopause and you have always been very thin, for example—it is worth seeing your doctor before problems develop. You may be able to have a bone-density scan to determine whether preventative steps are necessary.

Living with osteoporosis

People with osteoporosis are usually prescribed drugs to promote normal bone growth. Women will be offered hormone replacement therapy.

Your doctor will also discuss safe ways that you can exercise. Weight-bearing exercise is normally recommended, but you should avoid prolonged or strenuous activity. If you have osteoporosis, walking a mile or more a day is probably the best exercise since it minimizes any jarring to the bones. You are also likely to benefit from gentle back-strengthening exercises to improve your posture—stooping puts additional pressure on the spine and may increase the risk of spinal fractures. Exercise such as tai chi, which helps to improve balance and posture, may also be helpful because it can reduce the likelihood of injury from falls.

People with osteoporosis need about 1200mg of calcium a day; your doctor may recommend supplements of calcium and vitamin D to ensure that you get the right amount. Having a calcium-rich diet (see pages 88–9) is also important.

Help to reduce the risk of fractures by making sure that your home is safe: check for trailing cords or loose carpets that could cause a fall.

Doing yoga or breathing exercises can help you to manage stress. Bone-building minerals such as magnesium can be depleted by hormones produced when you are under pressure.

First Aid for Fractures

Fractures need emergency treatment—go to the local Accident and Emergency department, or call the emergency services. Fractured bones should be kept as still as possible, and it is essential that the injured person does not move if there is damage to the back or neck.

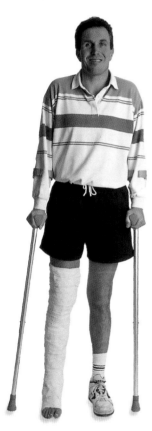

A broken leg will normally be encased in a plaster or resin cast while the bone heals and knits together.

Arm fractures

A fracture in the arm or collarbone can be very painful. The area may appear deformed and the person will not be able to move it. There is likely to be bruising and there may also be bleeding.

The injured person can usually walk, and can be taken to hospital by car, but it is important to keep the injured part as stable as possible—placing the arm in a sling (see right) will help. If the fracture is open, apply clean padding to either side of the bone and cover with a sterile dressing. Don't give the person anything to eat or drink since a general anesthetic may be needed.

Leg fractures

Fractures in the lower limbs are more serious than those in the arm, and you will need to call an ambulance for immediate assistance. If the thighbone has been fractured, there may be severe internal bleeding, which can lead to shock.

Do not move the person, but try to make him or her more comfortable: place padding such as rolled-up towels on either side of the leg, with the other leg alongside to help keep it still. You can bandage the legs together or gently hold the injured leg until help arrives. Cover the person with a blanket, but do not give any food or drink.

Making a sling

An arm sling is used for a fracture in the lower arm; it supports the forearm, hand, and fingers across the chest. To make a sling, you need a large triangular-shaped bandage. If you do not have access to a first-aid box, you can improvise by cutting up a clean sheet.

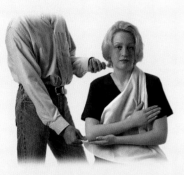

2 Lift the lower end of the bandage over the injured arm as the person continues to support it.

1 Help the person to hold the injured arm across the chest, and ask him or her to support the elbow in the palm of the uninjured hand. Place the bandage down the uninjured side of the body, as shown.

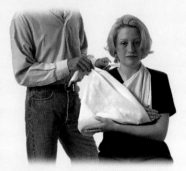

3 Tie both ends together, near the collarbone. Check that the hand and wrist are slightly higher than the elbow. Tuck or pin the edge of the bandage by the elbow.

Speeding Healing

Complementary therapies can be a useful adjunct to orthodox medical treatment for a fracture. They can help with the distress and shock that accompany the initial injury. Some remedies may soothe bruising and encourage the bones to knit together.

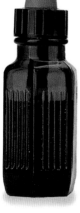

Instant help

The homeopathic remedy arnica can help to counteract the shock of the initial injury. Homeopaths recommend taking the remedy every ten minutes for the first hour, then three times a day thereafter to help soothe bruising. Placing a few drops of the Rescue Remedy—flower essences preserved in brandy—on the tongue as needed can help with feelings of panic and upset.

Further action

Homeopathic remedies, which are based on plants and other natural substances, can be used to help the broken bone to mend. Symphytum is usually recommended, so long as the bone has been correctly aligned.

Once the plaster cast has been removed, herbalists recommend applying comfrey, which is also known as "knitbone." Simply crush some fresh leaves and apply to the skin above the affected bone. Diluted thyme, rosemary, or marjoram essential oils can also be applied to the skin to encourage healing and soothe pain, but check that these oils are suitable for you. It is also a good idea to increase your intake of good bone foods—such as calcium-rich milk and cheese—while healing takes place.

Natural remedies such as comfrey leaves and flower remedies can be used to promote healing alongside orthodox forms of treatment.

Your Joints

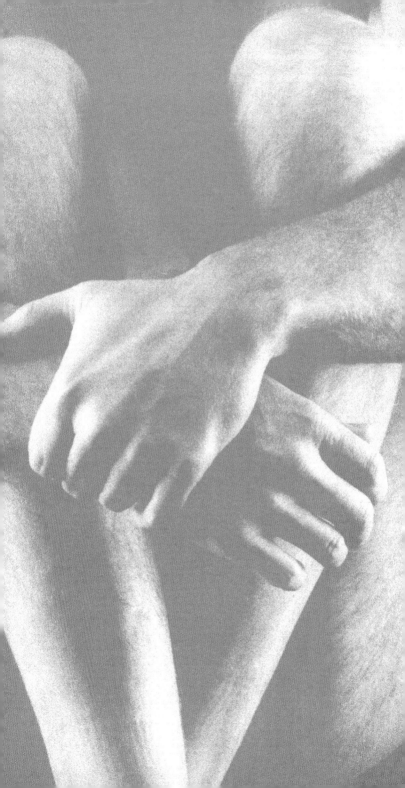

Keeping Mobile

Our joints tend to become stiffer as we grow older. Regular exercise keeps them flexible, and also strengthens the muscles and ligaments that stabilize them. In addition, exercise can help to minimize the effects of arthritis and other disorders.

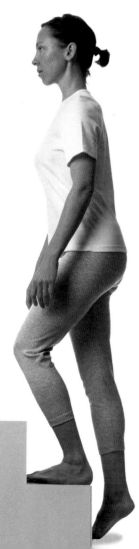

Improving flexibility

Any exercise can be beneficial to your joints, provided that you do it correctly. However, activities that encourage a range of movement are particularly good for the joints.

You should include some form of flexibility exercise in your fitness program. Yoga and tai chi are especially good, but aerobics and other fitness classes also include some flexibility work. Swimming and even activities such as housework can help to improve your suppleness.

Whatever type of exercise you do, make sure that you are using the correct techniques. Even gentle forms of exercise can cause injury if the movements are performed incorrectly or without proper attention to your alignment.

Seek advice from a qualified teacher if you are unsure about your technique. If you feel a twinge or pain in any joint while exercising, stop what you are doing immediately—it is much better to be overcautious than to risk an injury. If you feel the

Try to remain aware of your body at all times. Move in a relaxed, graceful way.

same pain next time you do the exercise, talk to your fitness trainer or a doctor. Take any joint injury seriously: you may need to adapt or cut back on your exercise while it heals.

Protecting yourself

It is essential to warm up before starting any form of exercise. Brisk walking on the spot, followed by some gentle stretches, will help to prepare your muscles and joints for physical activity. As a general rule, you should always keep your elbows and knees slightly bent; if you hold them rigid, they are more vulnerable to strain.

Be aware of your posture at all times. Standing up straight places minimum strain on the joints in your neck, back, hips, and knees. Losing any excess weight will also help your joints to work efficiently, and will reduce your risk of developing osteoarthritis as you age.

Ideally you should move each joint through its full range of movements every day. Avoid holding one position for extended periods: get up and stretch out or walk around if you are working at a desk, watching TV, or traveling.

Yoga is one of the best exercises there is for improving suppleness.

Preventing knee strain

Knee problems can often be avoided if you follow some basic safety precautions.

❶ Do not bend the knees too far—if they are extending farther than your toes, they are vulnerable to strain.

❷ Keep your knees facing forward, in the same direction as the toes: if they are twisted, sudden movements may cause damage.

❸ If you are running, do not stop suddenly; slow to a jog and then a walk.

❹ Keep the knees warm and protect them from damp and cold.

❺ If one knee is injured, do not overuse the other to compensate.

Eating for Healthy Joints

What you eat can play a major role in maintaining healthy joints. Following a well-balanced diet that includes plenty of oily fish, fruits, vegetables, and nuts may help prevent problems arising in later life. Diet may also assist in alleviating some of the symptoms of arthritis and other joint disorders.

Oily fish

Salmon, mackerel, herring, tuna, trout, and sardines are all good sources of essential fatty acids, which contain natural anti-inflammatory substances. Eating oily fish will help to keep your joints working well and has many other health benefits, too. Vegetarians can obtain fatty acids from nuts, seeds (especially linseeds), and whole grains.

Omega-3 oils can also be obtained from supplements. Taking a daily supplement—the usual recommended dose is 750mg—is worth considering if you find it hard to include enough oily fish in your diet. Supplements may even be a better way of obtaining these oils if you suffer from gout, since eating oily fish can encourage a build-up of uric acid in the joints.

Essential antioxidants

People who eat a diet that is low in the trace mineral selenium and in vitamins A, C and E may increase their risk of joint problems in later life.

You can get selenium from fish and shellfish, meat, whole grains, cereals, and eggs. If you eat a good variety of fruits and vegetables, you will

Water is the main constituent of synovial fluid, which lubricates the joints. Drink plenty of water every day to help your joints stay healthy.

obtain a wide range of vitamins. The best way to boost your intake of vitamin A is to eat liver (but not during pregnancy). Alternatively, orange and yellow fruits and vegetables—such as carrots, apricots, mangoes, and sweet potatoes—contain betacarotene, which the body converts to vitamin A. Citrus fruits, red and yellow bell peppers, kiwi fruit, cabbage, and Brussels sprouts are good sources of vitamin C, and vitamin E is found in olive oil, nuts, seeds, avocados, and beans.

What to avoid

Eating excessive amounts of red meat and highly processed foods can lead to a build-up of acid in the body, which is associated with gout and arthritic symptoms. Drinking large amounts of coffee, tea, and alcohol also has a negative effect, so you should keep your consumption moderate.

Extra help

If you do a lot of exercise, such as running, or you are experiencing stiffness or pain in the joints, it is worth asking your doctor about taking the supplement glucosamine. Glucosamine has proven anti-inflammatory effects, and research suggests that it helps to build new cartilage and enhance joint function. Another cartilage-building substance, chondroitin, can be taken with it. The usual recommended dose is 750mg, twice a day.

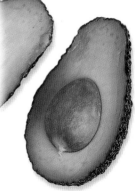

Following a healthy, balanced diet will reduce the risk of joint problems developing. Oily fish, whole grains, eggs, and avocados all bring vital nutrients to the body.

Injuries

Joint injuries can be very painful, and they may take several months to heal. The bones that form the joint may become displaced—dislocation—or there may be damage to the tough ligaments that hold the bones together.

Dislocation

Dislocation occurs when a twisting or wrenching action pulls a bone out of its normal position in a joint. A fracture can occur at the same time, and the surrounding ligaments may tear.

The fingers and shoulders are the most common joints to be dislocated. Dislocation is very painful, and the pain increases if the joint is moved. There is usually deformity and swelling around the joint, and there may be bruising.

If you dislocate a joint, you need immediate medical attention. An X-ray may be done to check for signs of a fracture. If there is no fracture, the affected bone can usually be manipulated back into position. Pain-killers and sedatives may be given while this is being done. The joint is then immobilized for several weeks, and you may need physiotherapy when you start using it. Dislocation can weaken the joint, making it prone to further problems. Sometimes surgery may be carried out to help stabilize it.

Sprains and torn ligaments

It is easy to overstretch or tear the ligaments in a joint, particularly those of the knee or ankle. Minor

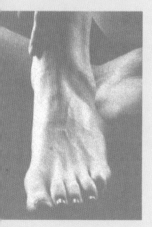

The ankle is vulnerable to sprains. You can easily tear a ligament simply by twisting the joint slightly as you step off a curb.

Shoulder dislocation

Dislocation occurs when one of the bones in a joint is wrenched out of place. It can usually be restored to position, but this can be painful and should be attempted only by a doctor.

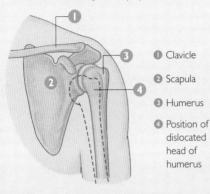

❶ Clavicle

❷ Scapula

❸ Humerus

❹ Position of dislocated head of humerus

Frozen shoulder

Frozen shoulder is very painful, and movement is restricted. Symptoms can develop over several weeks and may last for months.

Frozen shoulder can occur as the result of an injury, but there is often no obvious cause. The pain can be excruciating and is often worse at night. It lessens over time, but the shoulder becomes increasingly stiff. Symptoms are relieved by painkillers and anti-inflammatory drugs. In severe cases, a corticosteroid may be injected into the joint. Physiotherapy can often be helpful.

tears, known as sprains, often occur if the joint is twisted awkwardly as the result of a fall or during sports activity. They are particularly likely to affect the ankle. Damage can also occur if the joint is overworked, or if you do not warm up properly before exercising.

A damaged ligament causes pain that increases on moving. If movement feels excruciatingly painful, you may have ruptured the ligament and should seek immediate medical advice, because this can cause dislocation.

Minor sprains can easily be treated at home (see pages 118–19), and they usually heal fully within weeks. If the damage is more serious, physiotherapy may be needed. Occasionally the ligament is damaged so badly that it does not heal and needs to be surgically replaced—usually with a nearby tendon.

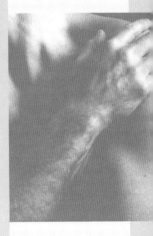

Bursitis and Torn Knee Cartilage

Bursitis

The bursae are fluid-filled sacs located around the joints. They serve to reduce friction where ligaments or muscles move over the bone. A bursa can become inflamed if it is placed under excessive or repeated pressure. It then becomes swollen and painful, and may feel hot to the touch. The swelling can limit movement, and the problem may take anything from between a couple of days to several months to heal.

Bursitis most commonly affects the knees, but it can also develop in the elbow or in other joints. It may be the result of an injury or excessive use, such as prolonged kneeling. The condition can also be associated with other joint problems such as rheumatoid arthritis.

The usual treatment is to rest the joint and to take anti-inflammatory painkillers. Applying ice-packs to the affected area can also help to soothe the inflammation.

Bursitis is often known as "housemaid's knee," but can occur in other joints of the body as well.

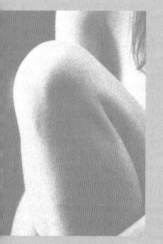

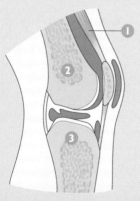

The bursae

There are ten bursae around the knee, which is the joint most likely to be affected by bursitis. If you have to kneel a lot, placing a rubber mat under your knees can help to prevent bursitis or stop it getting worse.

❶ Inflamed bursae

❷ Thighbone

❸ Shinbone

If the swelling persists, a doctor may use a needle to drain away the fluid; corticosteroids can then be injected into the area to prevent recurrence. Occasionally the bursa may need to be surgically removed, and antibiotics will be prescribed if it becomes infected.

Torn knee cartilage

Two cartilage disks—called menisci—act as shock absorbers between the thighbone and shinbone. These pads can become torn if the leg is suddenly twisted, as may occur in a footballing injury. The menisci are subject to wear and tear, and injury is more common in later life.

A sharp pain is often felt when the injury occurs, and you may also hear a tearing noise. Swelling develops within hours and movement is restricted. It can be difficult to put your weight on the affected leg.

Cartilage problems are serious and need prompt medical attention. An MRI scan may be done to assess the damage, and an X-ray may also be carried out to check whether there has been any injury to the bones.

The usual treatment is to rest the joint for at least two weeks, but those affected may never regain their ability to extend the leg fully. The knee is prone to further injury once the cartilage has torn, and there is a greater risk of developing osteoarthritis in the affected joint later on.

In severe cases, the cartilage may need to be surgically repaired. Most people regain movement within three weeks of surgery, but they may then need physiotherapy to help them improve mobility in the joint.

Torn knee ligament

The bones of the knee are kept in position by the tough medial ligament and the cruciate ligaments. Torn knee ligaments are a common sports injury, from which the knee joint never fully recovers.

❶ Torn medial ligament

❷ Torn cruciate ligaments

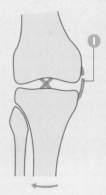

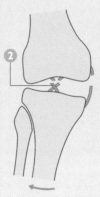

Arthritis

Arthritis is a general term covering a group of diseases affecting the joints. All of them cause pain, stiffness, and swelling. Most forms of arthritis cannot be cured, but the symptoms can be managed by drugs, diet, and exercise. Older people are most likely to suffer from arthritis, but younger people can be affected, too.

Osteoarthritis

Osteoarthritis is the most common form of arthritis. It usually affects those over the age of 60, although it can sometimes develop in younger people as well. In an osteoarthritic joint, excessive wear and tear erodes the protective cartilage that covers the ends of the bones. Tiny out-growths of bone (called osteophytes) form at the edges of the joint.

Many older people develop arthritic symptoms in the fingers. Doing regular hand exercises can help to reduce attacks.

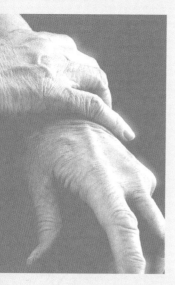

These changes cause pain and soreness, which worsen when the joint is used. There is usually swelling around the area, and movement is restricted. The joint may crack when moved. These symptoms can flare up and then go away for long periods. They often worsen as the disease progresses.

The hips, knees, spine, and fingers are most likely to be affected, but osteoarthritis can affect any joint. When it affects the spine, it is known as spondylosis (see *page 55*). It is more likely to occur if the joint has been under repeated stress, as the result of overuse or frequent injury.

Being overweight can increase your risk of developing the disease, and it can also run in families. Most people develop osteoarthritis to some degree by the time they are 70, but not everyone has symptoms. Women frequently experience more pain and stiffness than men.

Osteoarthritis is diagnosed by means of blood tests and X-rays. Symptoms can be relieved by non-steroidal anti-inflammatory drugs, such as ibuprofen or paracetamol. A corticosteroid may also be injected into the affected joint. Your doctor will give you advice on exercises that you can do to maintain mobility in the joint.

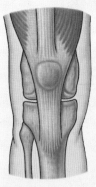

Osteoarthritis causes permanent damage to the bones, so early treatment is essential.

Joint Replacement

If a joint is damaged by a disease such as arthritis, it can be surgically removed and replaced with an artificial one. This operation is only carried out when other methods to relieve symptoms have been unsuccessful.

Hips are the most common joint to be replaced. The top of the thighbone is removed and an artificial ball and stem is inserted in its place. It fits snugly into a new cup socket inserted into the pelvis.

The new parts can be cemented into position. Alternatively the parts can be made from a porous material into which new bone tissue can grow and develop, holding the new joint firmly in place.

Recovery after uncemented procedure can take several months. The patient has to limit their activities while the new bone attaches itself to the new parts, and he or she may experience thigh pain while this is happening.

Most people who have a cemented joint recover within two to three weeks. However, there is a risk that particles of the cement may break off, causing inflammation. Also, if further surgery is necessary, it can be more complicated.

Older, less active people are usually given cemented replacements because of the quicker recovery time. Younger people are often given uncemented joints because they are more likely to need another joint replacement. Most artificial hip joints last 15-20 years.

Other Forms of Arthritis

Rheumatoid arthritis is a painful condition that is linked to a problem in the immune system. It gets worse over time and can increase your risk of osteoporosis and other disorders. Other less common forms of arthritis include gout and septic arthritis.

Site of septic arthritis

In septic arthritis, the protective membrane surrounding the joint becomes inflamed, and pus can accumulate within it. The pus may be drawn out with a needle (a process known as aspiration), and the joint needs to be rested for healing to take place.

❶ Pus

❷ Thickened synovial membrane

❸ Cartilage

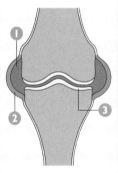

Rheumatoid arthritis

Rheumatoid arthritis is a progressive condition that starts with pain and stiffness in the joints. Over time, the pain increases and the joints become swollen, while small nodules can appear under the skin. Rheumatoid arthritis can damage the bones, so early treatment is essential.

The causes of the disease are not fully known, but it is thought that the body's immune system starts to attack the tissue and bone in the joints. It is more common in women and usually affects those over 40. The fingers, wrists, knees, and shoulders are most likely to be affected.

There is no cure for the disease, but it can be slowed down by anti-rheumatic drugs. These can have serious side-effects, so sufferers need to be monitored through frequent blood tests. Gentle exercises are recommended in between attacks to help maintain joint mobility. As with osteoarthritis (see pages 112–13), a joint can be injected with corticosteroids to relieve pain.

Septic arthritis

Septic arthritis is a bacterial infection of the joint. The bacterium can enter the joint by way of a nearby open wound, or it may originate from elsewhere in the body. Symptoms include fever, swelling and redness around the joint, pain, and reduced mobility. Early treatment is essential.

Fluid may be drawn from the joint and checked for signs of infection. Septic arthritis is treated with antibiotics, given intravenously for several weeks. Non-steroidal anti-inflammatory drugs may also be prescribed.

Gout

Gout occurs when there is a build-up of the waste product uric acid in the toe or other joints. Symptoms, including pain and inflammation, tend to flare up and then recede. The condition often runs in families, but being overweight, drinking too much alcohol, or eating large amounts of meat or processed foods can increase your risk. Uric-acid levels can be checked by blood tests and by analyzing fluid drawn from the affected joint. Symptoms can be relieved with non-steroidal anti-inflammatories, corticosteroids, or an anti-gout drug. Other drugs may be given to prevent uric-acid levels from building up.

Reactive arthritis

Reactive arthritis occurs after an infection in the genital tract. An abnormal response by the immune system causes swelling and the build-up of pus in the joints. The underlying cause needs to be treated with antibiotics, and non-steroidal anti-inflammatories help relieve joint symptoms. Most people recover fully.

The knees go through a lot of wear and tear in our lives, and they are commonly affected by arthritis. A knee replacement operation may be recommended if drugs do not ease your symptoms.

Other Joint Disorders

You should consult a doctor if you experience increasing pain in a joint that has no obvious cause, or if your child develops an unexplained pain or limp. A physical examination and X-rays can usually determine the cause.

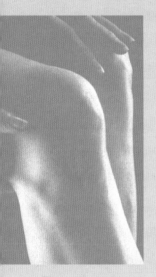

The cartilage around the kneecap is affected in chondromalacia, making bending one or both knees painful.

Chondromalacia

Chondromalacia is a condition affecting the cartilage around the kneecap. Actions that involve straightening and then bending the leg—such as going up and down stairs—cause severe pain, and the joint may feel stiff after a long period of sitting. Usually just one knee is affected, but sometimes it occurs in both knees.

Chondromalacia mostly affects adolescent girls, and it sometimes runs in families. The exact cause is not known, but it may be the result of the thigh muscles pulling the kneecap in an awkward direction. It is most likely to develop in girls who have suffered injuries in the joint or who play a lot of sport.

The condition is diagnosed by a physical examination and confirmed by X-rays. Pain-killers, non-steroidal anti-inflammatories, and ice-packs all help to relieve symptoms. Sufferers are also advised to wear a knee support and rest the joint as much as possible. Once the pain has lifted, a physiotherapist may recommend exercises to strengthen the ligaments around the joints and the thigh muscles to prevent further problems.

Osteochondritis dissecans

In osteochondritis dissecans, the blood supply to part of a joint is cut off. The affected bone and cartilage may die, but remain inside the joint. This causes pain and swelling that worsens after physical activity. The joint (commonly the knee) may also lock without apparent reason. If part of the joint has died, it will be surgically removed. Otherwise, wearing a knee support and avoiding strenuous exercise will help relieve symptoms.

Systemic lupus erythematosus

In this disease, the immune system starts to attack some of the body's tissues. It causes inflammation and pain in the joints, similar to the symptoms of arthritis, and the person may also get a fever and fatigue. An itchy red rash may develop, often over the nose and cheeks, and some people experience hair loss. Lupus is more likely to affect women than men.

The condition is diagnosed by a blood test. There is no cure, but corticosteroid or, in severe cases, immunosuppressant drugs ease symptoms. Physiotherapy can also help joint problems.

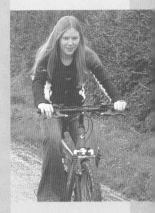

Children with Osgood-Schlatter's disease must avoid strenuous exercise until they are over 14.

Osgood-Schlatter's

A painful swelling develops just under the knee in this condition. It is most likely to affect teenage boys who do a lot of exercise.

Osgood-Schlatter's occurs when the quad muscles of the thigh pull excessively on the tendon attached to the shinbone. This causes pain that gets worse after exercise, limping, and restricted motion. Rest usually resolves the problem, but sometimes the joint needs to be immobilized in a plaster cast for several weeks.

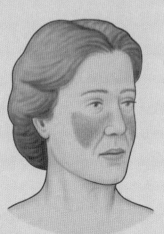

A butterfly-shaped rash can spread over the nose and cheeks in the auto-immune disease systemic lupus erythematosus.

First Aid for Sprains

In a sprain, the ligaments surrounding the joint become over-stretched and can suffer a minor tear. These injuries can usually be treated at home. However, if there is severe pain or if you think that a bone may be broken, seek medical advice straightaway. You should see your doctor if self-treatment does not help.

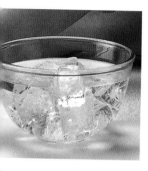

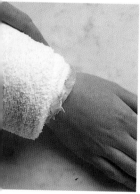

Top: **Ice cubes can be used to soak a compress or make an ice-pack.**

Above: **Thick padding placed over the sprain area will help any swelling to go down.**

Immediate action

Sprain treatment involves a standard first-aid procedure of rest, ice, compression, and elevation —known as RICE for short.

Rest Help the injured person into a comfortable position, moving the affected joint as little as possible. Place the joint on a soft support such as a cushion, or in your lap, so that it stays steady while you treat it. Do not place any weight on the joint for 24–48 hours.

Ice Apply a cold compress or an ice-pack to the joint. If using an ice-pack, do not apply ice directly to the skin: wrap the pack (or a bag of frozen vegetables) in a clean towel or dishcloth first. You should apply ice to the area five or six times over the next 24 hours, for no more than ten minutes at a time. This will help to minimize any bruising and swelling.

Compression Surround the joint with a thick layer of padding to apply even pressure to the area. This also helps to reduce swelling. Secure the padding with a soft elastic bandage, but make sure it is not too tight.

Elevation Raise the joint above the level of the heart to help excess fluid drain away.

Complementary help

Arnica is a homeopathic remedy that can prevent bruising: apply the ointment over unbroken skin before bandaging. Comfrey cream and distilled witchhazel can also be helpful. If using a compress, you can add a herbal decoction or essential oils such as lavender, eucalyptus, or rosemary to the water. Dilute it in a carrier oil or in full-fat milk.

Comfrey's other name of "knitbone" attests to its use in bone and joint injuries, and comfrey cream may be applied to help heal sprains.

Severe injuries

If the pain is so severe that you cannot move the joint, or if it gets worse after 24 hours, see a doctor. He or she may need to immobilize the area with a splint or bandage, and may prescribe strong pain-killers. An X-ray may be done to check that the bones are not broken.

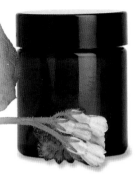

How to make a compress

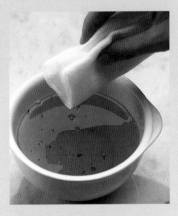

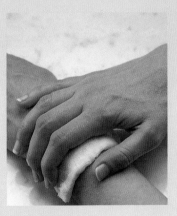

❶ Fill a bowl with very cold water— add a few ice cubes if you have some to hand. You can add diluted essential oils or a herbal decoction (as shown above) at this stage. Drop a clean cloth into the water.

❷ Remove the cloth from the water and wring it out. Apply to the area for about ten minutes. Keep the cloth cold by returning it to the water every so often. Reapply the compress every few hours for a day or so.

Living with Arthritis

Drugs can help to control arthritic symptoms, but there are also plenty of natural methods that you can use to help yourself. Research shows that exercise is highly effective in relieving arthritic symptoms, but changing your diet may also help.

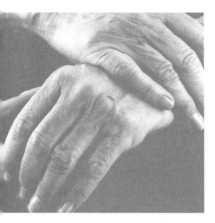

Gentle activity is the best way to reduce stiffness in the fingers and other joints. Clench the fists and then open out the hands regularly.

Keeping active

Exercise can increase your mobility, reduce the severity of arthritis attacks, and lift your mood. In general, people with arthritis benefit from doing specific exercises to mobilize the joints, as well as aerobic exercise to improve strength and fitness. Brisk walking, cycling, swimming, tai chi, yoga, and Pilates can all be valuable.

Ask your doctor to refer you to a physiotherapist for advice on exercising safely.

As a rule, you should rest joints when they are painful and exercise them when the symptoms have receded. Whatever exercise you choose to do, it is essential that you warm up properly before exercising: it may help if you apply a warm compress to joints before exercising, and a cold one (or an ice-pack wrapped in a towel) immediately afterward.

Diet and supplements

If you are overweight, ask your doctor to refer you to a dietician for help. Carrying excess weight places unnecessary strain on your joints and can exacerbate arthritic symptoms.

People with arthritis benefit from eating a healthy, balanced diet that includes plenty of fruit, vegetables, whole grains, fish, and white meat. Eating oily fish once or twice a week can help to relieve painful inflammation in the joints; one study found that rheumatoid arthritis sufferers dramatically improved their symptoms by eating 7 ounces of salmon a day. However, oily fish can exacerbate symptoms in people with gout (see page 115). Walnuts, green tea, and fresh ginger also have anti-inflammatory properties.

Some people find that arthritic symptoms worsen if they eat certain foods: in particular, red meat, eggs, tomatoes, potatoes, eggplants, or bell peppers. It may be worth keeping a note of what you eat so that you can pinpoint possible triggers and then avoid them.

Supplements of glucosamine and chondroitin (see page 107) can benefit people with arthritis, particularly those who suffer from osteoarthritis.

Natural relief

Heat treatment can help to relieve pain and stiffness: apply towels soaked in hot water to the affected area, take a warm bath or shower, or use a hot-water bottle wrapped in a towel or a gel pack heated in the oven or microwave. Some people benefit more from applying an ice pack. Experiment to see which works best for you.

You may also gain relief from complementary therapies like acupuncture, homeopathy, gentle massage, or aromatherapy. Using specially adapted tools, such as thick-handled cutlery or long-handled tongs, may make daily life easier.

In daily life, you should avoid holding any one position for a prolonged period: if you are watching TV, for example, stand up and walk around at regular intervals. You could also consider getting a rocking chair: rocking can help to improve your flexibility and strengthen the knees.

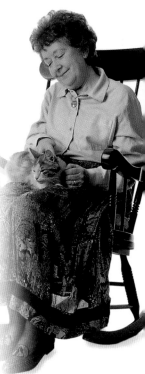

Useful Therapies for Joint Problems

If you suffer from painful joints, a physiotherapist can give you advice on useful exercises to do. He or she may also use massage and manipulation to help restore mobility. Many people find that complementary therapies such as chiropractic or acupuncture help: ask your doctor about the suitability of these therapies for you.

Massage

Massaging around a joint helps to warm sore areas and encourages the removal of toxins. Shiatsu (*shown below*) can also help joint problems; pressure is used to improve the flow of healing energy through the area. If you have arthritis, choose a therapist used to treating your condition: massage can cause harm if it is done incorrectly.

Manipulation therapies

Manipulation combined with exercise can help to speed healing of a sprained joint. Chiropractors and osteopaths use slightly different techniques, but both aim to free the joints and improve mobility. They also use massage to relax the surrounding tissues, which can go into spasm after an injury. Their therapies may be of benefit after the first 24–48 hours, during which time the RICE procedure should be used (*see page 118*).

Osteopathy and chiropractic can also help people with osteoarthritis: one study reported in the *British Medical Journal* in 1991 found that these therapies produced better results than physiotherapy. Joint manipulation is not recommended for people with rheumatoid arthritis, but stretching and trigger-point techniques can be helpful.

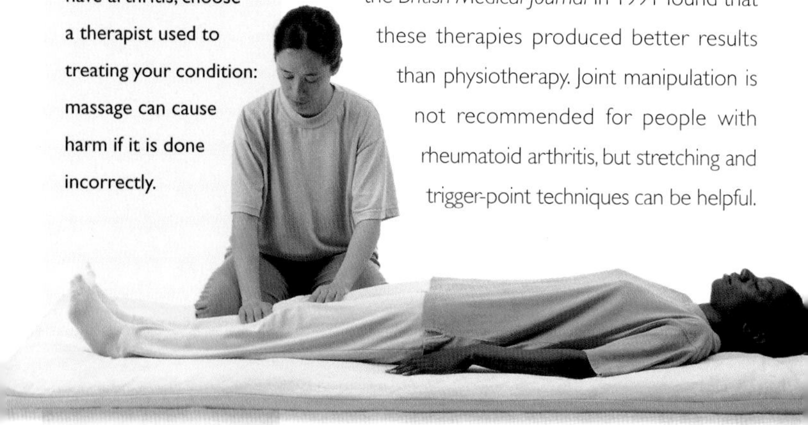

Preventive therapies

Maintaining good posture will help relieve stress on the joints; it will also ensure that you move in a way that minimizes any pain. The Alexander Technique is one of the best ways to improve your posture: classes are usually given on a one-to-one basis so that you can focus on your individual needs.

Practicing yoga or the Chinese healing exercise tai chi can also improve the way that you hold yourself. In addition, these exercises can reduce stiffness and keep joints mobile. Make sure you seek out an experienced teacher who is aware of your particular problems: certain yoga postures are not suitable for people with arthritis.

Relaxation therapies

Living with frequent pain can be distressing, but you may be able to reduce your symptoms through relaxation. Some people find that pain worsens when they are stressed because their breathing becomes too quick and shallow. Deep breathing exercises, yoga, and tai chi can all help you to manage stress and anxiety. Hypnotherapy may also help you to manage your pain better and you should ask your doctor if he or she can recommend a reputable practitioner.

Herbal treatments

There are several homeopathic remedies used to relieve arthritis, including apis and calc. carb; see an experienced practitioner for advice on which remedy is most suitable for you. Western herbalists may recommend turmeric or Chinese skullcap, which have anti-inflammatory properties.

Acupuncture

Acupuncture has been shown to help relieve pain, and it can also reduce inflammation.

Several studies have found this therapy to be helpful in relieving the symptoms of people with osteoarthritis and rheumatoid arthritis. Acupuncturists may stimulate particular points on the body by inserting a fine needle, or by moxibustion. In this gentle, warming technique, a stick of the herb moxa (mugwort) is lit and held over certain points to stimulate them.

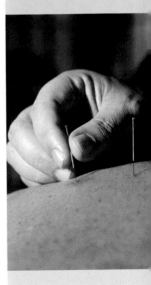

Preventing Knee Strain

Knee strain is very common—you can easily cause damage to the ligaments by twisting the joint. These Chinese exercises work well as a preventative routine, and they can help if you have a minor injury that is healing. If your knee hurts or is swollen, or if you are unused to exercise, talk to your doctor first. Do not let the knee extend farther than the toes when squatting.

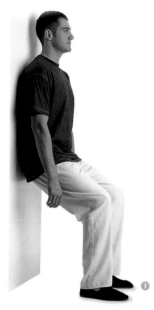

2 If you find step 1 easy, move your feet closer to the wall. Squat down so that there is an angle of 80° between thighs and shins, and let your hips move away from the wall slightly. Take care that your knees do not push farther than the toes —if they do, you are too close to the wall. Hold the position until you can feel your thighs working, then come up slowly. Repeat two or three times.

Backward Squat

1 Stand tall, about 18 inches from a wall, with your feet hip-distance apart. Lean your back against the wall, and squat so that your thighs are at an angle of 90° to your shins—or as close as you can comfortably get. Breathe evenly in this position until you feel a warm tingling in the thighs. Come up slowly.

Wide Squat

1 Stand in a wide stance, with your feet facing forward and knees slightly bent. Your arms should hang down by your sides, shoulders relaxed. Your spine should be straight, with the head in line with it—imagine that a cord is attached to the top of your head and is pulling you upright.

2 Squat down, making sure that your knees do not extend farther than your toes. Bend forward from the waist, keeping your back straight. Clench your fists and bring them in front of your abdomen.

3 Hold the squat for a few moments, then straighten up, keeping a bend in the legs. Breathe in and out slowly. Repeat the squat two more times, holding for a little longer each time. Keep the shoulders relaxed at all times.

125

Releasing Stiff Shoulders

These exercises are good to do if you work on a computer, or if you have stiffness in the shoulders due to arthritis. Try to do them at least once a day; two or three times daily is ideal. Take a few moments before you start to stand in a comfortable way—check the posture pointers on page 18—and breathe deeply to help relax the body. Make slow, smooth movements, and do not push your shoulders farther than they will comfortably go.

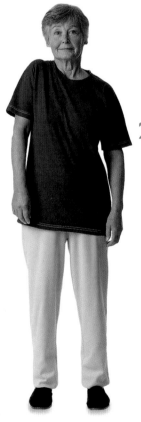

Shoulder Circle

1 Move your right shoulder as if tracing a circle with the tip. Make five counterclockwise circles, then five clockwise ones. Do not let the shoulder tense up; keep the arm hanging down throughout.

2 Do the same with the left shoulder. As you become more practiced, gradually increase the number of circles to a maximum of ten.

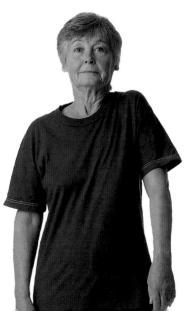

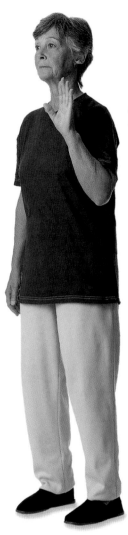

Hand Press

1 Raise your left hand in front of the left shoulder, keeping the elbow dropped and the arm and shoulder relaxed.

2 Slowly press forwards with your hand, straightening the arm as if pushing something away from you. Bring it back and repeat up to ten times. Do the same on the other side.

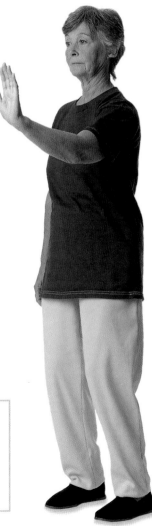

HELPFUL HINT

The best way to foster a smooth, relaxed movement is by breathing out when you push the arm away and breathing in as you draw it back again. Try to develop a smooth rhythm as you move the arm back and forth.

Arm Raise and Swing

I Raise your arms above your head. Bring your palms together and interlace the fingers, then turn the hands so that your palms are facing upward. Make sure that your shoulders remain relaxed and loose as you extend the arms upward. Keep the back straight and the head and neck erect, but not tense.

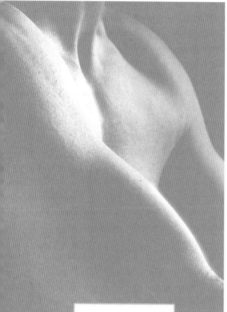

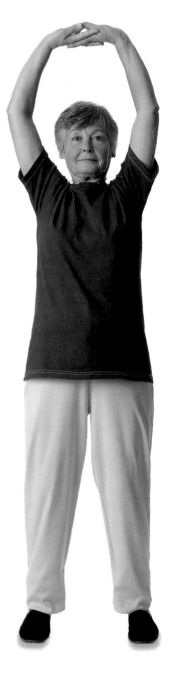

HELPFUL HINT

Take care that you don't draw the elbows back farther than the ears as you raise the arms, as this will cause tension in the shoulders.

2 Slowly lower the hands behind the head, resting your interlaced fingers on the back of the skull and keeping your elbows up. Now raise them up and back down again, up to ten times. You may like to synchronize the arm lifts with your breathing: inhale as you lift up and exhale as you drop the hands back down again.

3 Bring your arms back down by your sides. Then slowly swing one arm back as you swing the other one forward. Do 10–20 swings, moving the arms briskly and rhythmically, and breathing normally throughout. Don't forget to keep the shoulders dropped and relaxed at all times.

Freeing Frozen Shoulder

Frozen shoulder causes stiffness and severely limits movement. It may be due to an injury or muscle strain, but often no cause can be found. These exercises may help you to regain mobility in the joint, but they should be done only under the advice of your medical practitioner. Go gently and do not push the shoulder too far. You may need to leave some exercises out until your mobility improves.

Forward Arm Raise

1 Stand tall with a straight back, feet shoulder-distance apart and knees slightly bent. Hold a broom handle in front of you as shown.

2 Bring your arms out in front of you and then up above your head—or as far as you can easily manage. Keep your arms straight—but not locked—as you lift up the handle.

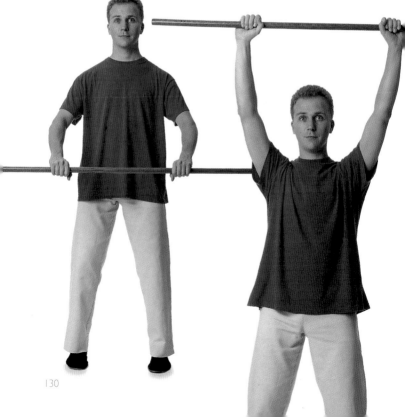

3 Now lower the arms back to your starting position. Repeat several times, up to a maximum of ten repetitions. Gradually increase the speed of the raises, but keep a steady rhythm. Keep breathing evenly throughout, and make sure your shoulders remain relaxed.

Backward Arm Raise

1 Now hold the broom handle behind your back, in a comfortable position. Do not grasp it too firmly; keep your hands relaxed.

2 Lift the handle out and as far upward as you can comfortably manage. Keep your back straight as you do this and stop if you feel any strain. Lower the handle back to the original position. Repeat, doing a maximum of ten repetitions.

Broom-Handle Twist

1 Hold the handle in front of you, at chest height. Your elbows should be comfortably bent. Slowly turn from the waist to your left, keeping your head in line with your spine and your feet and knees facing forward.

2 Now turn to the right, going as far as feels comfortable. Continue turning from side to side, up to a maximum of ten times. Gradually increase the speed of your turns, but try to keep a steady rhythm. Make sure that your shoulders remain relaxed throughout, and that you keep breathing normally.

Back Reach

Reach behind your back, bending the elbow so that you can place the hand as high as possible—you may not be able to raise it very far at first. Repeat on the other side. Do up to ten repetitions, keeping the shoulders relaxed.

Elbow Lift

Stand tall, but relaxed. Raise the affected elbow, lifting it up as high as possible. Touch the back of your neck with your hand, keeping the back straight. Lower the arm and repeat up to ten times.

Elbow Reach

❶ Raise your arms and bend the elbows. Interlink your fingers behind your neck and relax the shoulders.

❷ Bring your elbows as far back as comfortably possible. Repeat this closing and opening action up to ten times.

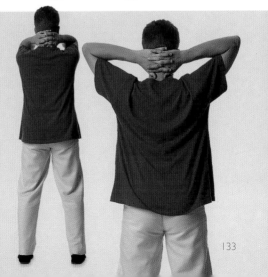

133

Clasped Hand Raise

1 Stand up straight, with your knees slightly bent and your arms by your sides. Bring your arms behind your back. Rest your hands just above the buttocks, palms facing outward and fingers interlaced. Check that your shoulders are loose and relaxed.

2 Slide your hands up the back, as high as they will comfortably go. Ensure that you do not tense the shoulders as you raise your hands. Return to the starting position, and repeat up to ten times.

Upward Reach

Stand about 12 inches away from a wall or a ladder. Place your hand at shoulder level—or as close to it as you can manage—and hold for a moment or two. Then raise your arm a little higher, and hold again. Repeat a few more times, going a little higher each time, if you can.

HELPFUL HINT

You can use any tall, sturdy object for this exercise—such as a bookcase if you are indoors, or a tree if you are outside.

Preventing and Easing Arthritis

Arthritic joints benefit from gentle activity to keep them mobile. However, you should not try to exercise them when they are painful and inflamed. In between flare-ups, you can practice these exercises daily. You may find that some techniques, such as the squat (*see page 141, step 2*), feel difficult when you first start—if necessary, leave them out until you build up greater flexibility.

Finger Stretch

❶ Clasp a pencil firmly in your fist.
❷ Place your palm on a flat surface, such as a table, to straighten it. Repeat several times.

Taking care of yourself

When you are living with a chronic condition such as arthritis, you need to make sure that you are exercising in a way that is beneficial. Talk to your doctor before starting these exercises to ensure they are suitable for your particular condition. If you find that any of the exercises increases your pain, stop and consult your doctor.

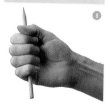

Wrist Flex

Press your palms together, then use one hand to press the other wrist joint back. Repeat on the other side. Do this several times, increasing the speed and pressure. Then try holding a beanbag or light dumbbell as you bend and straighten the wrist.

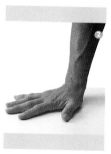

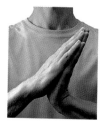

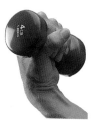

Consider learning tai chi: this gentle form of exercise involves continuous whole-body movements, which can help to prevent and improve arthritic symptoms as well as boost your general health. Tai chi will also help you to practice these exercises in a relaxed, focused way. Ask your doctor for his or her advice, then seek out remedial classes with an experienced teacher.

Elbow Opening

1 Stand tall, but relaxed. Make your hands into fists. Raise them and rest the knuckles on the top of your shoulders.

2 Open your arms out wide, so that they are about 12 inches away from your thighs. Return the fists to the shoulders and repeat three times.

Shoulder Loosening

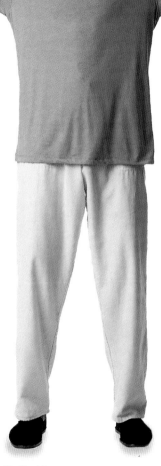

1 Stand tall, with your arms by your sides. Your knees should be hip-distance apart and slightly bent.

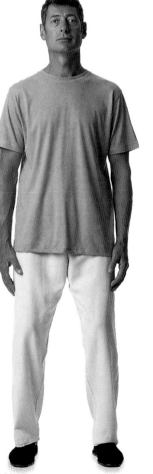

2 Stretch your arms out to the sides, keeping the elbows slightly bent. Bring them up to shoulder level, or as close as you can manage.

You can do this exercise at various intervals throughout the day. Gradually build up the number of repetitions that you do—the movements will become much easier with practice.

Ankle Mobilizer

Sit upright in a chair, feet flat on the floor. Raise one leg: point your toes and then flex and straighten the foot a few times. Now rotate the foot, first in a clockwise direction, then in a counterclockwise direction. Repeat on the other side.

3 Continue raising the arms above your head, bringing the hands together in a prayer position if you can. Lower and repeat three times.

Shoulder Curling

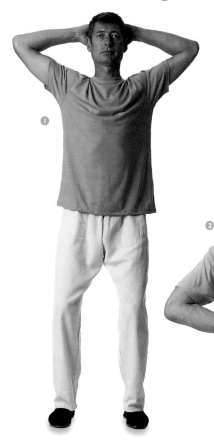

2 Lower your arms and bring your hands behind your back. Interlace your fingers again, palms pointing outward as shown. Bring your shoulders forward and toward the center of your body. Keep them relaxed and do not force the movement. These exercises help to increase the forward and backward mobility of the shoulders.

Stand tall, with your feet hip-distance apart and knees slightly bent. Raise your arms, bending the elbows so that you can rest your hands on the back of the head. Interlace your fingers. Now slowly draw back the elbows to open the shoulders. Do not let them tense up: keep them relaxed throughout the exercise.

Hip/Knee Releaser

1 Take a step forward with your right leg. Bend the right leg well and let the left one straighten. Place your hands on your hips. Draw the elbows back as you lean the upper body slightly forward. Hold this position for a few minutes, breathing normally. Take a step forward with the back leg, to resume the starting position. Then repeat the stretch on the other side.

HELPFUL HINT

Make sure the feet point in the same direction, and that your knees are aligned directly over them. Do not allow the knees to extend further than the toes.

2 Hold onto a sturdy chair for support. Squat down as far as feels comfortable for you (you may not be able to go very far). Use the power of your leg muscles to come up slowly, keeping your back straight.

Leg Swing

I Stand tall by a chair, holding onto it with the right hand. Bend the right knee slightly. Slowly swing the left leg forward, letting it straighten as you do so.

HELPFUL HINT

Take your leg as high as you can without causing any discomfort. Try to develop a smooth, steady rhythm as you swing the leg backward and forward.

2 Now swing the leg behind you, bending the knee. Repeat the forward–backward action up to ten times, keeping a steady rhythm and breathing normally. Change legs and do the same on the other side.

Your
Muscles

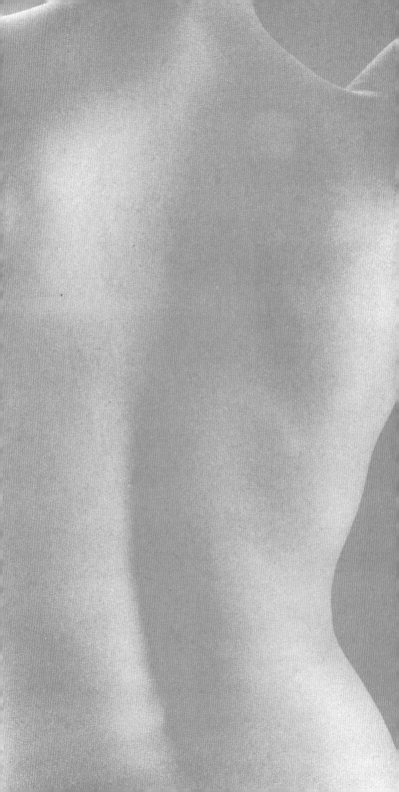

Healthy Muscles

Regular exercise builds strong, toned muscles, and it helps to keep the heart fit and healthy. Most of us do not do enough exercise, but it is easy to increase the amount you do. Try walking or cycling to the stores instead of driving, taking the stairs instead of the elevator, or volunteering to walk somebody's dog.

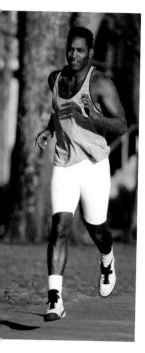

When you can continue running for more than 20 minutes at a time, your body will start to burn up the calories stored as fat.

Building your fitness

There are three aspects to fitness: strength, stamina, and suppleness. Stamina is the ability to exercise continuously for a long period; you have to exercise for at least 20 minutes before you are in a position to lose weight, for example.

You need a certain amount of stamina in order to do aerobic exercise. This is any activity that leaves you slightly out of breath, raises your heart rate, and works up a sweat. When these things are happening, oxygen is being burned at a higher rate inside the body, thereby using up calories. Good forms of aerobic exercise include aerobics, fast walking or swimming, and running.

Strength-building exercises increase the power of the muscles. When you lift weights, for instance, the effort causes muscle fibers to break down. When these fibers repair themselves, they grow back stronger. Muscle tissue uses more calories to maintain itself than fat does: you may find that you put on weight if you build muscle, but you will be leaner and healthier.

Both aerobic and strength-building exercise can place a strain on the joints and muscles, so it is a good idea to do some suppleness exercise to keep

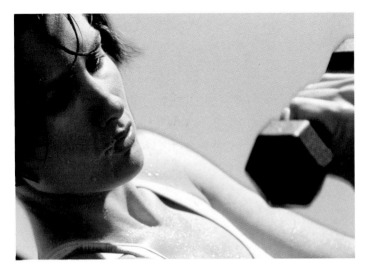

your joints, ligaments, and muscles in good shape. Suppleness is built by stretching the muscles so that they become more flexible and less likely to tear. Tai chi, yoga, and warm-up stretches all help to increase suppleness.

A sensible combination of these three forms of exercise is the best way to increase your fitness, lose excess weight, and guard against injury. You need to build your fitness slowly: see your doctor for advice on exercising safely.

Lifting weights helps to build strength and power in the muscles.

Increasingly sedentary lifestyles mean that most people in the West do not do enough exercise.

Why muscles ache

When we work our muscles in an unfamiliar way, they start to ache. This may be because lactic acid —a waste product—accumulates in the muscles. When we rest, the circulation works to flush out lactic acid. Gentle massage or having a hot bath or shower can help to boost the circulation and thus relieve aching. Strong muscles produce less lactic acid—so the fitter you are, the less you should ache after exercise. Doing warm-up and cool-down stretches will also help.

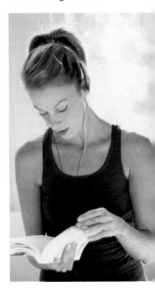

Fueling your Muscles

Eating the right foods and drinking plenty of water will ensure that you are getting enough energy to power your fitness program. Avoid smoking and drinking excess alcohol, since these will drain your energy and undermine your ability to exercise. Junk foods and too much sugar will also have a negative effect.

Drink plenty of water throughout the day, and especially before and after exercise, to make sure that you are properly hydrated.

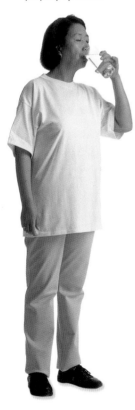

Eating for healthy muscles

Our muscles consist mostly of protein. You need to obtain about 2 ounces of this nutrient each day in order to give the muscles what they need for repair and renewal. This should not be difficult, because protein is a constituent of many foods: meat, poultry, fish, cheese, eggs, cereals, pulses, nuts, and potatoes are all good sources. A ½-pound portion of chicken is enough to supply your daily needs. Protein-rich foods should be eaten in moderation, however, since excess protein may put strain on your liver and kidneys.

Energy for the body

If you are doing a lot of exercise, you need to make sure that your diet is providing you with sufficient energy (calories). The best foods for energy are complex carbohydrates, such as bread, potatoes, rice, cereals, and pasta. These foods are broken down into glucose, which the body uses to power the muscles.

Instant energy-boosters—which may be useful just before or during an exercise session—include bananas, dates, raisins, and dried apricots.

Water works

Make sure that you drink plenty of water (at least eight to ten glasses a day). Water is almost like fuel—you get tired and have less stamina if you are not completely hydrated. Try to sip water during exercise; if you feel thirsty, you are already dehydrated. And be sure to drink plenty of water after an exercise session to replace fluid lost through perspiration.

Relaxing the muscles

Stress and anxiety can cause us to hold ourselves in a semi-permanent state of muscle tension—this uses up unnecessary energy and makes our joints and muscles more prone to injury.

Learning ways to relax is an essential part of keeping the muscles healthy. Yoga, tai chi, swimming, and relaxation techniques can all be helpful. Physical exercise also has a relaxing effect; the very act of moving your muscles releases built-up tension. Breathing deeply and steadily during exercise sessions also encourages relaxation.

A good night's sleep is another essential element of building your fitness. The body repairs tissue much faster during sleep, and even having a nap can help speed muscle repair.

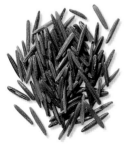

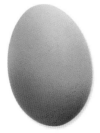

Protein is found in many foods, from meat and fish to cereals and eggs. It is an essential nutrient for the muscles, but it is easy to eat too much of it—stick to a moderate intake of protein-rich foods.

Muscle Squeeze and Release Exercise

Exercise can help you to relax more easily. However, it is also a good idea to learn specific relaxation techniques that you can use on a daily basis. Over time, these can help you become more aware of your body, so that you will notice when tension starts to build up and can then take steps to release it.

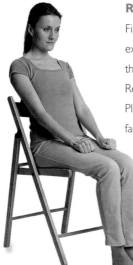

If you need a quick relaxer during the day, sit down and spend five minutes doing the relaxation exercise described on page 149. Start with the toes and feet, and work gradually up the body. Sit quietly, breathing evenly, for a few moments afterward.

Relaxation position

Find a comfortable position for the relaxation exercise. If possible, lie on your back (*below*)—in this position, you can let yourself sink into the floor. Rest your head on a soft pillow for extra comfort. Place your arms out to the sides, with your palms facing upward, or rest them on your abdomen—whichever feels right to you. Let your feet flop out to the sides. You can place a pillow under your knees if extending them straight out puts any pressure on your lower back. Try to bring your sitting bones slightly forward and upward before you start—this helps to get your spine into its optimum position. It is also a good idea to cover yourself with a light blanket, since lying in any one position for a long period causes your body temperature to drop.

Relaxation Exercise

This exercise involves contracting the muscles of your body, area by area. As you release them, tension will drain out of your body. Before you start, take a few moments to make sure that you are in a comfortable position. Take a few deep breaths to help relax the body before you start.

1 Bring your attention to your feet. Squeeze the toes into the ball of your foot and hold for a few moments. Release. Then press your heels downward, so that you feel the stretch in your calf. Hold this for a few moments, then release.

2 Now work up to your thighs and buttocks. Squeeze the muscles in and hold. Then release the tension.

3 Focus on your lower abdomen. Breathe in and then, as you exhale, let the abdomen sink toward the floor. Repeat.

4 Curl your shoulders forward and inward. Hold for a moment or two, then let them drop back to the floor as you breathe out. Now bring them up toward your ears using a shrugging action. Hold and release.

5 Clench your fists, feeling the stretch in your forearms. Hold and then relax them. Repeat.

6 Drop your chin to bring it closer to your chest. Again, do not strain as you do this. Hold, and then release the tension.

7 Now move up to the face. Purse your lips, then relax them. Grin like a Cheshire cat, then let your mouth drop back into its natural position. Frown, and then relax again. Squeeze your eyelids together, hold and then gently release the tension.

8 Your body should be feeling relaxed and soft at this point. Let your breathing find its natural rhythm as you stay in the relaxation position for 5–10 minutes.

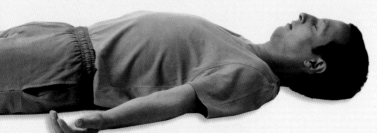

Strengthening the Pelvic Floor

Both men and women can benefit from strengthening the muscles of the pelvic floor. Do each of the exercises described here until you feel slightly fatigued. The first exercise is the most important, and can also be done sitting down or standing up—try to practice it two or three times a day. It is important for women to strengthen the pelvic floor during pregnancy and after childbirth, because the muscles can become stretched and this may increase the risk of urinary incontinence in later life. If you are pregnant, do only the first exercise; after 30 weeks, do it sitting up, since lying on your back can reduce the blood supply to the baby.

Pelvic Squeeze and Release

1 Lie on the floor and relax. Breathe in and tighten the muscles of the pelvic floor (the same action that you use if you want to interrupt the flow when urinating).

2 Breathing out, release the pelvic muscles. Repeat until you feel mildly fatigued—over time, you will be able to increase the number of repetitions that you do.

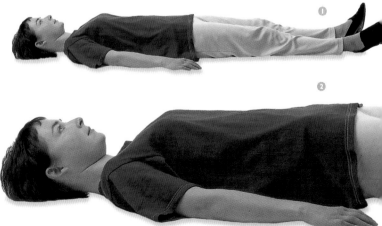

Hip Raise

1 Bend your knees so that you can
place your feet flat on the floor.
Breathe in and lift your lower back
off the floor, tensing your buttocks
and pelvic-floor muscles.

2 Breathe out and lower yourself
slowly down to the floor again.
Take a deep breath and relax
the body. Repeat this exercise as
often as you like, but stop when
you feel tired.

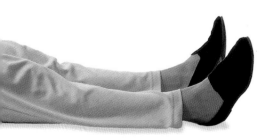

Muscle Injuries

It is easy to injure a muscle if you perform a sudden awkward movement, if you do strenuous exercise after a long period of inactivity, or if you exercise when the muscles are cold. Warming up will help to protect you from injury.

Cramp

Cramp is a painful muscle contraction that can last several minutes. Any muscle can be affected, but it often occurs in the foot, calf, or hand. Cramp often strikes during exercise, especially if the muscles are cold before you start. It is usually due to the build-up of lactic acid inside the muscle, but it could also be the result of drinking too little water and becoming dehydrated.

Cramp can also occur when a muscle is held in one position for too long, as seen in writer's cramp or at night during sleep. Occasionally, the problem is connected to a deficiency of calcium or salt, both of which are needed for muscle contraction. Gently stretching or rubbing the affected area usually helps to relieve the discomfort. However, if you experience frequent cramp, see your doctor: cramp can occasionally be a sign of narrowed arteries or diabetes. Older people often experience repeated cramps at night. A doctor may prescribe quinine to help with this.

Cramp is most likely to occur during exercise, particularly if you have not warmed up properly. Dehydration is another possible cause.

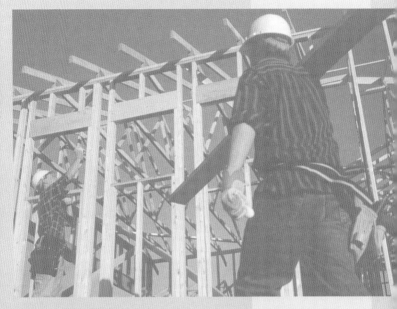

Lifting something that
is too heavy for you can
strain the muscles of
the abdomen and back.

Strained (pulled) muscle

Muscle fibers can become overstretched or torn
if excessive demand is placed upon them—
for example, if you perform a sudden, jerking
movement or if you engage in a bout of strenuous
and unfamiliar activity. Most athletes will strain a
muscle at some point.

The surrounding fibers go into spasm to
prevent further movement and this can feel very
painful. Other symptoms include swelling and a
small amount of bruising. Self-treatment is usually
all that is needed (see *pages 160–1*), and the pain
should subside within a day or two. Over-the-
counter non-steroidal anti-inflammatories can help
to relieve pain and swelling.

Ruptured muscle

**A torn muscle can
take weeks to heal,
and physiotherapy may
be needed to help you
rebuild its strength.**

If you suffer a severe
strain, you may need
an X-ray to check for
fractures. The area will
become swollen and
bruised within hours,
and there may be
considerable pain.
Sometimes the whole
muscle can rupture: if
this is the case, you may
see two bulges with a
gap in the middle.

Muscle and Tendon Problems

One of the most frequent problems to affect the muscles and tendons is inflammation due to overuse. This can take many forms, from repetitive strain injury to tennis elbow. Another common condition is restless leg syndrome, which affects one in eight people.

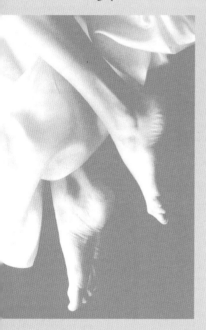

Restless leg syndrome is a deep sensation of restlessness that is relieved when you move the legs. It often strikes at night, and can seriously interrupt sleep.

Restless leg syndrome

Restless leg syndrome is an uncomfortable restlessness in the leg muscles: people experience it as a burning, tickling, prickling, or aching sensation. It usually comes on at night.

Nobody knows why this syndrome affects some people, although it is occasionally linked to diabetes or anemia. There is no known cure, but stretching or warming the muscle can help, as can acupuncture. In severe cases, anti-convulsants, may improve symptoms.

Repetitive strain injury

RSI, as this syndrome is commonly known, is muscle or tendon strain caused by frequent, repetitive movements involving the arm and hand. Symptoms may include a dull aching, heaviness, cramp, pins and needles, or severe pain. These usually affect the hand, wrist, and forearm, although they can also occur in the neck and shoulder.

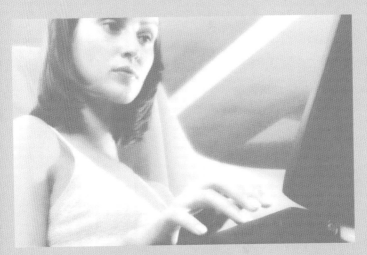

People who work on keyboards or production lines are prone to RSI, and research shows that it is more common in those suffering from stress. If it is left untreated, it may lead to permanent damage, so see your doctor as soon as possible.

Your doctor may recommend that you wear a wrist brace and that changes are made to your work station. You may be referred to a physiotherapist for specialist exercises that can prevent the condition getting worse. Placing a hot-water bottle wrapped in a towel on the area can be soothing, and anti-inflammatory drugs may help.

See your doctor if you notice that your hands, wrists or shoulders start to ache after working on a keyboard. Treatment is more effective if RSI is caught early on.

Safety at work

If you work at a computer, make sure that your work station is correctly set up for you. Your employer should help you to do this (see also pages 22–3).

❶ Forearms They should be roughly horizontal and resting on the desk.

❷ Wrists Use a wrist rest to keep your wrists in line with your hands.

❸ Fingers Do not clutch the mouse or press the keys too hard.

❹ Breaks Rest the fingers every 20 minutes or so.

Other Tendon Problems

Tendinitis and tenosynovitis

Tendinitis is inflammation of the tendon. It is usually due to overuse, but may sometimes be the result of an infection. One of the most common sites to be affected is the Achilles tendon in the back of the heel. Inflammation here may be due to a sports injury—hill runners are prone to problems in the Achilles tendon—or the result of ill-fitting shoes that dig in at the heel. The tendons in the wrist are also frequently affected, resulting in the condition known as repetitive strain injury (see page 154).

Some tendons, such as those of the wrist and ankle, are surrounded by a protective sheath that secretes synovial fluid to reduce friction. This sheath can become inflamed—a condition known as tenosynovitis. This often occurs at the same time as tendinitis. It is usually the result of an injury, but it can also affect people with rheumatoid arthritis.

If tenosynovitis affects a finger, the tendon can become locked when the finger is flexed. It can then suddenly release with a jerky movement—this condition is known as trigger finger.

Symptoms of both tendinitis and tenosynvitis include swelling, pain, and restricted movement in the affected area. There may be a tender lump over the tendon and sometimes the skin can feel hot.

The treatment for tendinitis and tenosynovitis is the same as that for muscle strain: rest and non-steroidal anti-inflammatory drugs. Antibiotics will be given if the underlying cause is an infection.

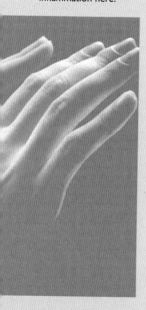

The tendons in the hand lie just beneath the skin, which makes them vulnerable to injury. People who do a lot of repetitive movements with their fingers, such as pianists, computer operators, or factory workers, may develop inflammation here.

Tennis elbow

Tennis elbow is caused by repeated gripping and twisting actions, such as those involved in using a screwdriver.

In this condition, the tendon attaching the muscles of the forearm to the outer elbow becomes inflamed. The area feels tender, and movement is restricted. Golfer's elbow is similar, but affects the inside of the elbow. The joint needs to be rested, and anti-inflammatories and physiotherapy can help.

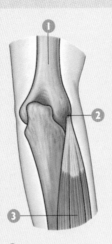

❶ Humerus

❷ Area of tenderness at elbow joint

❸ Muscle of the forearm

Ruptured tendon

Tendons are made of tough fibrous tissue, but they can tear if the muscle to which they are attached contracts violently – this usually occurs as a result of lifting something heavy or playing sports. The Achilles tendon is the one most likely to rupture completely. The hamstrings behind the knee, or the patella tendon which links the quadriceps muscles of the thigh, can also be subject to tearing.

If a tendon ruptures, you may feel a ripping sensation. Other symptoms include severe pain, restricted movement, and swelling. Non-steroidal anti-inflammatories are the usual treatment. If the Achilles tendon is affected, the area may need to be immobilized in a cast while healing takes place. Occasionally surgery may be needed.

Carpal tunnel syndrome

The carpal tunnel in the wrist is a narrow space through which the median nerve passes. If the wrist tendons become inflamed, they may cause a narrowing of the tunnel and place pressure on the nerve.

Symptoms include pain and aching in the hand, particularly around the thumb, index, and middle finger and the palm. There may also be tingling and weakness. A wrist splint and anti-inflammatories can help. Carpal tunnel syndrome often affects people who use their fingers a lot, such as pianists.

❶ Area affected by carpal tunnel syndrome

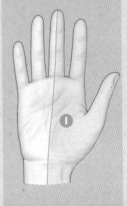

Muscle Disorders

Most muscle problems are short-term, although chronic problems can sometimes develop. These include fibromyalgia, which involves widespread muscle pain, and myasthenia gravis, an immune disorder that affects the nerves.

Wry neck

In torticollis, the muscles of the neck contract involuntarily, causing the head to be held in an abnormal position. The problem usually comes on overnight, and it is much more likely to affect women than men. Stress can be a factor.

❶ Sternomastoid muscle

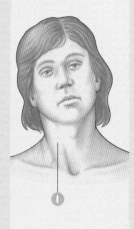

Torticollis

In this condition, which is also known as wry neck, muscle spasm in the neck causes the head to tilt or twist to one side. This produces pain, stiffness and sometimes trembling. In adults, torticollis is frequently the result of assuming an awkward position in sleep. It is occasionally linked to cervical spondylosis (osteoarthritis in the upper back and neck, see page 55). Torticollis can also occur in newborn babies after a difficult delivery: the most likely cause is an interruption in the blood supply to the muscles.

In babies, several sessions of physiotherapy will be needed to help maneuver the neck into the correct position. Treatment for adults involves pain-killers, heat, and massage. Your doctor may also recommend that you wear a neck collar. In most cases the problem clears up within two weeks. However, in persistent cases a relaxant may need to be injected into the muscle.

Nervous tic

A tic is an unintentional, repeated contraction of a muscle. The cause is usually psychological. Tics commonly take the form of rapid blinking or the twitching of the facial muscles, such as those around the mouth. Sometimes there may be an involuntary jerking of the neck, or shrugging of the shoulders. Tics are common in children, and they usually clear up with maturity, although they can sometimes develop after a head injury or stroke. Psychological therapies can help to relieve underlying stress factors, and sometimes anti-anxiety drugs may be prescribed.

Fibromyalgia

People affected by this condition experience aching in the muscles, particularly those of the upper back, abdomen, and legs. The base of the skull and the area between the shoulder plains may feel particularly sore. The person in question may also feel generally fatigued and suffer frequent headaches. Those suffering from fibromyalgia are often prone to depression and anxiety.

There is no proven treatment for fibromyalgia, but your doctor may refer you to a physiotherapist for massage, heat, and ultrasound treatment. A course of low-dose anti-depressants may also be recommended.

Infections and tumors

Infections do not usually spread to the muscles, but a viral infection such as flu can cause muscular aches. Bacterial infections (for example, tetanus) can cause the muscles to go into spasm.

Very occasionally, tumors can develop in the muscle – these are called myosarcomas. Fibroids are non-cancerous tumors that develop in the womb. They affect one in three women and often cause no symptoms. Sometimes fibroids may lead to abdominal pain and heavy periods, in which case they can be surgically removed.

Myasthenia gravis

In this disorder, the body produces antibodies that attack nerve endings in the muscles.

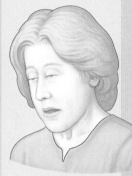

Myasthenia gravis stops the nerves from receiving instructions from the brain. The muscles fail to contract properly and become weak. The face and throat are most often affected, causing drooping eyelids, problems in eating, and slurred speech.

The problem can be linked to a tumor in the base of the neck. If so, the growth can be surgically removed. Otherwise drugs can be taken to improve the functioning of the nerves and reduce the production of antibodies.

Easing Muscle Pain

Most muscle problems get better with home treatment, but you should see your doctor if pain persists or is very severe. You can buy anti-inflammatories such as ibuprofen from the pharmacist to help relieve the pain of muscle strain.

When to see a doctor

• If symptoms do not start to improve within a couple of days.

• If swelling or pain starts to worsen.

• If cramp persists for longer than an hour, if you have a persistent leg cramp; or if you get cramp while walking.

• If you have other worrying symptoms such as fever, headache, numbness, or bruising.

• If pain is excruciating: you may have torn a cartilage or ligament, or fractured a bone.

• If widespread muscle pain occurs for no obvious reason.

Relieving cramp

To prevent cramp, do a daily routine of stretching and make sure that you drink lots of water before, during, and after exercise. If cramp strikes, gently stretch the muscle and then massage the affected area: this helps to stimulate the circulation and encourage the removal of lactic acid. You can do this in various ways, depending on the area that is affected by cramp.

Hand For cramp in the hand, keep pulling your fingers straight and massaging them until the discomfort wears off. Rub your hands together to bring heat to the area.

Leg If cramp strikes in the leg, ask a friend to massage it for you. To relieve cramp in the lower leg, lie down on the floor. Your helper should gently pull the lower leg straight while holding the knee in place. He or she should cup your heel in his or her hand, and then push the toes upward (toward the knee). Gently rub and massage the area once the initial spasm wears off.

Another way of stretching the muscle is to stand in front of a wall. Step back with the affected foot, then place your hands on the wall and lean forward. This should give you a good stretch in the lower leg.

Foot If cramp affects the foot, place it flat on the ground. Your helper should then lift up your toes and gently pull them straight. Rub the foot afterward, and put on some warm socks.

First aid for strains

Muscle strain should treated by the RICE method (Rest, Ice, Compression, and Elevation, see page 118) whenever possible. After the first 24 hours, applying a warm compress usually helps to relieve aching: use a clean cloth soaked in hot water, a hot-water bottle wrapped in a towel; or a gel pack heated in the oven or microwave.

Massaging the affected area can also be very soothing. Take a warm bath or shower first to help relax the muscles, then use gliding and kneading movements to work the affected area. Use the tips of your thumbs to release tension from tender spots. Ask a friend to do this for you if you cannot easily reach the muscle.

When to start moving

If your muscles are stiff and aching, give them a rest for two or three days. After this, start to resume normal activity: long rest periods are not advised because they may lead to the muscle fibers shortening.

Start to work the muscles gradually: resume normal activities and do a few minutes' exercise several times a day, stopping if you feel any pain. Gradually build up the amount of exercise that you do, until normal mobility returns. This can sometimes take weeks or months, depending on the severity of the problem.

Massage helps to break down muscle tension and increase blood flow to the affected area. To work stiff shoulders, bend the opposite arm across your chest and use your hand to massage the painful area. Support the elbow in your other hand.

Useful Therapies

Physiotherapists use a range of treatments to encourage healing of muscle problems. They tend to work with people who have serious injuries. If you have a minor problem that is taking a long time to heal, massage and other complementary therapies may be helpful.

Shiatsu

Eastern massage uses pressure to enhance the flow of energy along invisible pathways in the body.

Although the theory behind shiatsu is very different to that of Western massage, it can have similar effects—relaxing the muscles, releasing spasm, and improving flexibility.

Physiotherapy

Physiotherapists help to restore muscle strength and flexibility to normal after an injury. Treatment usually includes specialized exercises, which you can practice at home, and massage to relieve pain and muscular spasm.

Hydrotherapy treatment may be used. For this, the patient practices exercises in a heated pool: the water can support his or her weight and provide resistance for the muscles to work against. Ultrasound may be used to send heat to the tendons or muscles, which promotes healing.

You may need only one or two sessions of physiotherapy, or a long-term course may be recommended, depending on your problem.

Immediate treatment after an injury can stop the muscle going into spasm, and shorten the time healing takes.

162

Massage

Massage is an excellent way of relieving muscular pain and tension. It helps to release spasm, and improves the circulation of oxygen and nutrients to the soft tissues. The squeezing and pummeling that take place also help to stimulate the lymph system, which works to remove waste products such as lactic acid from the tissues.

Most therapists practice Swedish massage, which combines soothing strokes with deep pressure. Sports masseurs use similar techniques, but specialize in treating injuries. Aromatherapy massage is more gentle, and aromatic oils with specific healing properties are smoothed into the skin. Another form of massage is Rolfing. This uses vigorous techniques to unlock tension. It can be uncomfortable to undergo, but may help to reduce pain afterward. Massage should be started a few days after the injury, once the healing process has begun. It should not be given if there is swelling, bruising, or any fever.

Other therapies

Osteopaths work on the soft tissues to stretch out the muscle, which can be helpful after an injury. Chiropractors use similar techniques. Both types of therapist may treat any distortions in the spine and joints at the same time.

If a sports injury is slow to heal, acupuncture can be a good way of relieving discomfort. Moxibustion—in which a herb is burned on or just over certain points in the body—is a warming treatment that can also help to release muscle tension. Acupuncture may also ease the symptoms of fibromyalgia for short periods.

Techniques

Swedish massage involves various techniques to relax or stimulate the soft tissues. The overall effect is highly pleasurable.

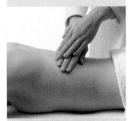

Gentle stroking helps to relax the muscles, and encourages the release of endorphins, the body's natural pain-killers.

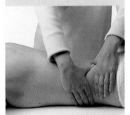

Kneading soothes tense muscles, breaks down spasm and increases blood flow to the area.

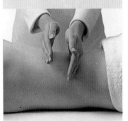

Percussion involves fast, rhythmic movements that stimulate the circulation.

Aiding Healing

Natural remedies can be a useful addition to your first-aid box. It is a good idea to get specific advice on remedies from a qualified practitioner. Some aromatherapy oils are not suitable for people with high blood pressure or those who are pregnant; some herbs can even have adverse effects. Always check that any remedy you take is suitable for you.

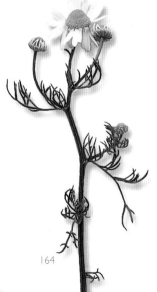

Rosemary is a warming herb that can ease aching and rheumatic muscles. Camomile is an anti-spasmodic that relieves tense muscles.

Homeopathy

Homeopathic remedies that may help with muscle problems include arnica, for bruising, pain after unfamiliar exercise, and help with shock after an injury. Ruta grav. can help if stiffness continues for longer than a day. Rhus tox. may be useful for restless leg syndrome and cramp,

Aromatherapy

Lavender or geranium can be massaged into the skin to help relieve cramp. Rosemary, camomile and lavender may relieve aching muscles if a few drops of essential oil are added to a warm bath or smoothed directly onto the affected area. Essential oils can also be added to the water for a hot compress. All aromatherapy oils should be diluted in a carrier oil, such as almond oil, before they are applied to the skin or added to bathwater.

Herbal remedies

Cramp bark is a traditional remedy for relaxing the muscles. Herbalists may recommend that you rub the ointment into the skin of the affected area. Distilled witchhazel is a gentle healer that can be added to a compress.

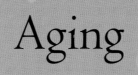

Aging

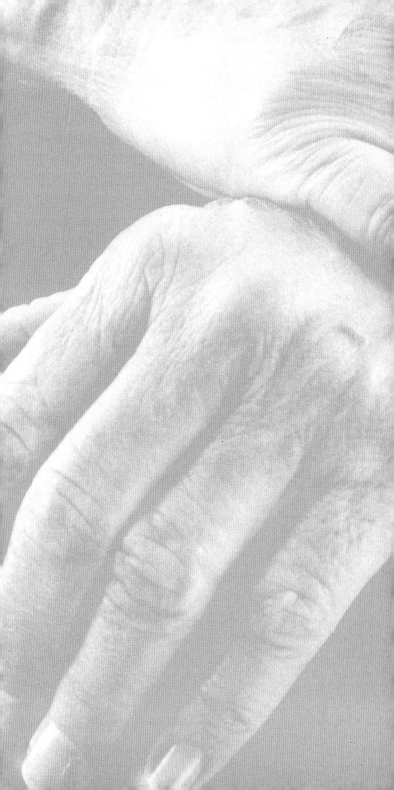

How We Age

These days we are living much longer than we used to. New medical discoveries and improved health care mean that most people in the West are living into their seventies and beyond. But longer life expectancy doesn't guarantee us good health. How fit and active we remain depends partly on our genes and partly on the way we live our lives.

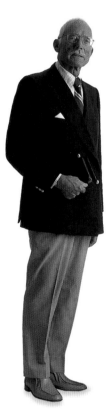

Having a sensible approach to exercise and diet will help you stay fit into your seventies, and beyond.

The aging process

We face health risks at every stage of life: a baby is particularly vulnerable to colds and other infections because the immune system is still developing, while working adults have a higher risk of experiencing stress and related problems.

In later life, the body naturally starts to slow down. Every part of us is affected: our skin loses its natural elasticity, the hair turns gray, our joints become less flexible, muscle strength declines, and the bones weaken. Daily life can become a little harder as our eyesight diminishes, our immune system weakens, and our digestion becomes less efficient. We are more likely to develop problems such as osteoarthritis (inflammation of the joints due to wear and tear, see *pages 55 and 112*), osteoporosis (loss of bone density, see *pages 56 and 94*), and cancer.

Staying healthy in later life

Aging is a natural process, and we will never be able to conquer it fully, but there is a great deal that we can do to increase our chances of living a healthy life for longer. Getting regular exercise and having a balanced diet are the two main

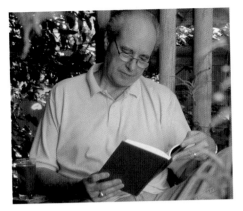

components of healthy living: they help the body to stay strong and active, and may prevent us succumbing to disease. If you smoke, giving up is the best thing you can do for your health: this will quickly reduce your risk of many serious diseases and will help your skin to look more youthful. Getting plenty of sleep and having regular health checks are also important.

Reading books that make you think or doing a daily crossword will help to keep your brain functioning well.

Yoga and meditation are proven to reduce stress and induce relaxation. They are suitable for people of all ages.

Mental health

As we grow older, our short-term memory can become less efficient and our ability to concentrate may be reduced. You can help to improve the long-term performance of your brain by keeping mentally active: doing a daily crossword, testing your memory, and stimulating your intellect by reading or learning a new language are all beneficial. Finding ways to reduce or manage stress is also important: practising yoga, tai chi, or relaxation exercises may help. Getting regular physical exercise also has a positive effect because it helps keep the circulation working well, ensuring that the brain receives the supply of oxygen and nutrients that it needs to stay healthy.

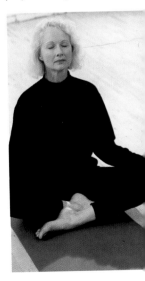

Healthy Weight, Healthy Life

Sedentary lifestyles and unhealthy diets mean that increasing numbers of us are overweight: more than 50 percent of Western adults are now carrying too much weight. But maintaining a healthy weight helps to reduce your risk of many diseases that can shorten life or reduce the quality of your lifestyle.

Opposite: **Keeping active in later life will help you maintain a healthy weight.**

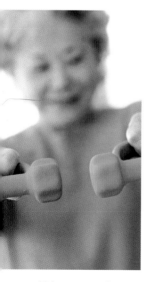

Make sure you choose exercise that is suitable for your level of fitness: your doctor can give you advice on this.

The right weight

Doctors use the body mass index (BMI) to assess whether or not you are a healthy weight. This index provides a good indication about the amount of body fat that you are carrying. You can use the simplified BMI (*opposite*) to check whether your weight is in the healthy range for your height. Be aware that the BMI is a rough guide only: if you are athletic, you may weigh more than is recommended, because muscle weighs more than fat, but you will still be healthy.

How excess weight is distributed around the body also affects your health. If you are apple-shaped—that is, you carry excess weight around the waist—you have a greater risk of heart and circulatory diseases than if you carry fat elsewhere in the body. Ideally, your waist measurement should be no more than 36 inches if you are a woman; 40 inches if you are a man.

Overweight or underweight

Being either overweight or underweight can increase your likelihood of getting certain diseases and also makes it hard for your body to function effectively. If you are underweight, you may be taking in insufficient nutrients to build healthy muscles and strong bones, thereby increasing your risk of osteoporosis. If you are overweight, you are placing unnecessary pressure on your joints and your internal organs. Diseases such as diabetes, osteoarthritis, and heart disease are all more likely.

Losing weight

The best way to achieve and maintain a healthy weight is by having a healthy diet and exercising. Fad diets often work in the short term, but most people regain the weight that they lose.

If you have health problems or are very overweight, discuss any plan to gain or lose weight with your doctor. To lose weight, exercise regularly —build up to at least three or four 30-minute sessions a week. Aim to lose about 4½–9 pounds a month; weight lost steadily is easier to keep off.

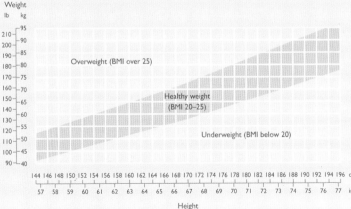

Body mass index

Locate your height and weight, and then find the point where they meet on the chart. This gives you some indication as to whether or not your weight is in the healthy range.

Weight
lb   kg

Overweight (BMI over 25)

Healthy weight
(BMI 20–25)

Underweight (BMI below 20)

210 — 95
200 — 90
190 — 85
180 — 80
170 — 75
160 — 70
150 — 65
140 — 60
130 — 55
120 — 50
110 — 45
100 —
90 — 40

144 146 148 150 152 154 156 158 160 162 164 166 168 170 172 174 176 178 180 182 184 186 188 190 192 194 196 cm

57 58 59 60 61 62 63 64 65 66 67 68 69 70 71 72 73 74 75 76 77 in

Height

A Healthy Diet

The food that you eat can change the way you look and feel, and it can help you live longer. Eating a balanced diet that contains plenty of fresh natural produce ensures that you are supplying your body with all the essential nutrients it needs.

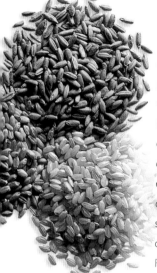

A balanced diet

A healthy diet is one that includes a wide variety of foods from the different food groups. These are carbohydrates, fruits and vegetables, proteins, dairy products, and fats.

Carbohydrates About one-third of your food intake each day should be made up of breads, cereals, rice, pasta, and potatoes. These carbohydrate foods are excellent sources of energy, and they also provide nutrients such as calcium, iron, and B vitamins. They are a good source of dietary fiber, which helps to keep the digestion healthy. Whole grains are best for this.

Fruits and vegetables You should eat five helpings of these foods every day. They are packed with the vitamins and minerals that we need to keep the

A healthy diet depends on eating the correct balance of foods, and not concentrating on one food group to the exclusion of others.

body healthy. Research shows that eating fruit and vegetables can help protect you from cancer and heart disease. They also contain fiber, which maintains healthy intestines and so helps to prevent bowel disease.

Protein foods Protein is needed for growth and repair of every part of the body—from the fingernails to the muscles. The best sources of protein are meat, poultry, fish, and tofu. Beans and pulses are also good protein foods, but they should be eaten with grains to maximize their nutritional value. Proteins should be eaten in moderation, making up just over 10 percent of your daily diet; excess protein can put a strain on the liver and kidneys.

Dairy products Milk, yogurt, and cheese are good sources of calcium, which is essential for healthy bones. They also provide protein. About 15 percent of your daily diet should consist of dairy foods. Low-fat versions are healthiest.

Fats and sugars You need some fat in your diet: it is an excellent source of energy, and it also helps the body absorb some vitamins. However, it should make up only about 8 percent of your daily food intake. Try to avoid fats that are solid at room temperature (such as butter and lard) as these increase cholesterol levels and, with it, the risk of heart disease. Replace them with unsaturated fats, such as olive and sunflower oil, which are much healthier. Sugary foods have little nutritional value, so you should eat them only sparingly.

Eating for Longevity

For optimum vitality, you need to eat plenty of vitamin-rich foods to boost the immune system. A healthy system will help fight off infections and disease, keeping you robust in later life. You may also want to include a few brain-boosters in your diet.

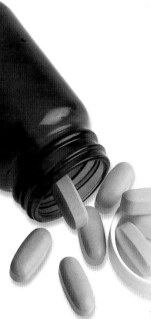

A healthy balanced diet should provide all the nutrients that your body needs. But a general vitamin and mineral supplement can be a useful safeguard, and your doctor may recommend B12 supplements to help boost the memory.

Essential nutrients

We become less active as we get older, so we generally need to eat less. But although we may need fewer calories, our requirements for many important vitamins and minerals increases.

Vitamins B6 and B12 The body's ability to absorb these nutrients is reduced with age, and increasing your intake of B12 may help to keep the memory working well. Try to include good food sources in your daily diet: these encompass pork, liver, and fish. Eggs, whole-grain cereals, brown rice, bananas, pulses, and yeast extract also provide B vitamins. If you notice that you are becoming more forgetful than before, discuss taking vitamin B12 supplements with your doctor.

Vitamin C This vitamin helps to strengthen the immune system and increases your absorption of iron. Citrus fruits, kiwi fruit, tomatoes, and broccoli are all good sources.

Calcium and vitamin D Your body needs these nutrients to build strong bones. Sunlight stimulates the body into making vitamin D, so spend at least 15 minutes a day outdoors. For calcium, eat dairy products, fish with edible bones, apricots, fortified orange juice, and baked beans. Combined supplements may be recommended for those at

Some research suggests that taking the herbal remedy ginkgo biloba may help to delay the development of Alzheimer's disease.

risk of osteoporosis, or elderly people who are housebound.

Vitamin E This helps keep the immune system healthy and is good for the skin, which becomes drier in older age. It may also help keep mental faculties sharp. Seeds, nuts, wheatgerm, wholemeal bread, and green vegetables all provide vitamin E.

Zinc and copper These minerals also help to strengthen the immune system and improve the body's healing powers. Zinc-rich foods include meat, liver, and pumpkin seeds. You can get copper from liver, kidney, nuts, and cocoa powder.

Nuts are valuable sources of vitamin E, copper, and potassium.

Other good foods

If you have high-blood pressure, increasing the amount of potassium-rich foods that you eat may help: they include bananas, nuts, tomatoes, and avocados. Cut down on salt; try using lemon juice, garlic, or mustard to pep up the taste of your meals instead.

Oily fish contains natural anti-inflammatories, which can help reduce joint pain. They may also reduce the risk of heart disease, strokes, and Alzheimer's disease. Talk to your doctor about taking supplements if you do not eat much fish.

We become less aware of the signs of thirst as we age, so older people often cut down on liquids. But you need plenty of fluids to stay healthy: drink at least 8–10 glasses of water a day.

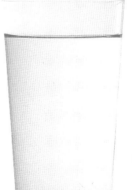

Sleep and Relaxation

Sleep is an important element of good health at any age. While we rest, our minds and bodies recover from the day's activities and carry out vital repairs. Lack of sleep can make us feel irritable and more prone to stress; it can also compromise the ability of the immune system to overcome illness. Most people need less sleep as they age, but you should still get enough sleep to wake up feeling refreshed.

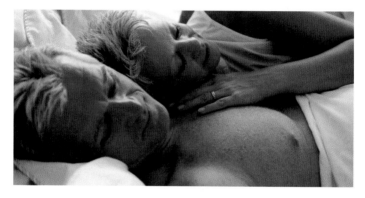

People need varying amounts of sleep—adults over the age of 60 often need only six hours' rest a night, supplemented by daytime naps.

Promoting good sleep

The key to good sleep is having a healthy lifestyle and establishing a good night-time routine. Doing regular exercise, not smoking, and having only moderate amounts of alcohol and caffeine can help you feel relaxed at bedtime.

If you have trouble sleeping, try to go to bed at the same time each night. Have a warm bath and a hot milky drink beforehand, to help get you in the mood for sleep. Make sure that you are comfortable and warm. If you do not drop off after 20 minutes, get up and go into another room until you feel sleepy. Practicing a relaxation exercise, such as those described opposite, may help.

Relaxation Exercises

When you are stressed, your muscles become tense, your breathing speeds up, and your heart beats faster. If stress is prolonged or frequent, these responses can be harmful to health: they may lead to sleep problems, anxiety, breathlessness, or palpitations. Relaxation techniques help you to breathe deeply, restoring calmness to mind and body. They can be practiced at any time.

1 Lie on your back and loosen any tight clothes. Rest your head on a soft cushion and close your eyes. Place your hands on your abdomen and let your feet flop out to the sides. Breathe in slowly and deeply. Breathe out in the same way.

2 Focus on your hands, and try to direct your breathing into the abdomen. As you breathe in, you should feel it rise up; as you breathe out, it should fall again. Continue breathing in this way for at least five minutes.

Variation

You can practice abdominal breathing sitting down.

Find a quiet place, close your eyes, and rest your hands on your thighs as you breathe deeply and steadily for five minutes. Alternatively, try silently repeating the word "Re-lax" as you breathe in and out. You can also practice the muscle squeeze and release exercise on pages 148–9.

Helpful Therapies

Natural therapies can be used in conjunction with orthodox medicine to treat illness and relieve symptoms. But they can be most effective as a form of preventative health care, to help you maintain well-being in body and mind. When choosing a complementary therapy, be guided by your own preferences. A therapy is more likely to work if you feel comfortable with it.

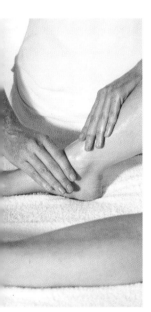

Most doctors see aromatherapy as no more than a relaxing therapy, but practitioners say that it can relieve many minor ailments and emotional disorders.

Time to talk

When you first see a complementary therapist, you usually spend a good deal of the session discussing your health and lifestyle. This gives you an opportunity to mention any ailments that you are experiencing—for example, constipation, fatigue or sleeplessness. Problems such as these may not seem important enough to report to your doctor, but they can make your life miserable. Complementary health therapies can provide a gentle and natural way of relieving such ailments, and so restoring good health.

Natural therapies can have powerful effects, so be sure to tell your doctor about any therapies you are considering; you also need to tell your practitioner about any medication or conventional treatment that you are having.

Massage

Having a weekly or fortnightly massage can be helpful if you find it hard to relax. Massage also helps to relieve minor aches and pains that could grow worse if left untreated.

Aromatherapists use aromatic plant oils in massage. The oils have a relaxing or energizing effect, and can help to reduce stress or relieve fatigue. Some have specific healing qualities—black pepper, for instance, is said to stimulate the appetite. Nobody knows quite how essential oils work, but it is thought that the aromas trigger a reaction in smell receptors in the nostrils, which then pass messages to the brain. The oils may also have an effect on nerve endings in the skin.

Acupuncture

Traditional acupuncture is based on the theory that energy flows along invisible channels in the body. When this energy flows freely, good health is maintained. However, when it is blocked, illness can result. Acupuncturists insert fine needles into certain points on the body to improve the flow of energy. The aim of treatment is to restore the body to its natural state of equilibrium. Specific complaints, such as digestion problems or back pain, can also be treated. Acupuncture is now accepted by many doctors as an effective therapy. A monthly treatment may help some people to maintain health in mind and body.

Reflexology

Reflexologists believe that every organ and part of the body is reflected in a point on the foot. They use massage and pressure to stimulate these points, with the aim of restoring health. Most people find reflexology treatment very relaxing A monthly session can be highly beneficial.

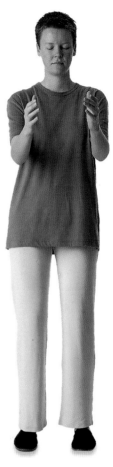

Chi kung (above) or yoga (left) are other good ways to stay healthy. Practiced regularly, they can improve your posture, aid the digestion, and improve breathing.

Quick Revitalizer

This exercise, practiced for generations in China, is a good way of relaxing and re-energizing the entire body. It can be done by almost anyone, no matter what their age or state of fitness, and is best performed daily. The main aim is to release tension from the body; it is also used to relieve headaches. Respect your limitations and slowly build up the number of swings that you do. Swing gently and do not bring the arms up too high. If you experience any dizziness, nausea, or other symptoms, stop what you are doing and rest. Check with a doctor if you have doubts about the suitability of this exercise (or any of those that follow) for you.

Stand upright. Tuck in your chin and your tailbone so that your spine and head are erect, but relaxed. Your feet should be hip-distance apart, facing forward. Bend your knees slightly and let your arms hang down naturally by your sides, leaving a little space under your armpits and keeping the elbows slightly bent. Relax your hands so that they are slightly curled and the fingers are apart. Relax your shoulders and abdomen, and take a few deep breaths.

3 Continue swinging your hands forward and backward, developing a relaxed, steady rhythm and breathing naturally. Do not try to coordinate your breathing with the arm swings. Swing until you feel energized, but not tired. Over time, you can gradually increase the number of swings that you do to 100. You may find it helpful to half-close your eyes and to focus on a point just below your navel as you swing.

2 Bring your hands forward and upward, but do not swing them any higher than your navel. Then let them swing behind you, bringing them no higher than your buttocks. This counts as one swing.

Variation

You can do this exercise sitting down, although the effects are not quite as powerful. Sit upright on a stool or a chair with no arms: your thighs should be at an almost 90° angle to the shins, and your feet should be hip-distance apart. Swing the arms backward and forward as described above.

Knocking at the Gate of Life

This is another quick Chinese exercise that is used to invigorate the body. It is said to promote longevity when practiced every day. The exercise works on the tan tien—an area just below the navel which, according to Chinese medicine, is the center of the body's energy. Two points on the front and back of the body—the Gates of Life—act as access points to the tan tien: these are stimulated in order to increase vitality and inner strength. The tapping actions and the waist turns also help massage the internal organs, improving the digestion and boosting the circulation. The exercise is best done early in the day, at least one hour after eating.

| Stand upright, with your spine and head erect, but relaxed. Place your feet wide apart, pointing forward. Bend the knees slightly. Relax your shoulders and let your arms hang down, slightly away from your body. Inhale deeply—breathing through your nostrils—and try to release any obvious tension from your muscles. Bring your hands into loose fists, without creating tension in the arms.

2 Rest the left fist on your lower abdomen (the Front Gate of Life). Place the right fist in the corresponding position on the back (the Back Gate of Life). Turn your upper body to the right, using your fists to strike these points gently as you do so.

3 Now turn the upper body to the left, letting your hands swing round and strike the opposite point. Keep turning and striking in this way, building up a natural rhythm and increasing your speed and the force of the taps. Breathe naturally through your nose as you swing. Continue the exercise until you feel energized and relaxed. Gradually build up the number of swings.

Invigorating Routine

This series of Chinese exercises encompasses self-massage and stretches, which can be done daily. They are suitable for anyone, including older people, but check with your doctor before you start.

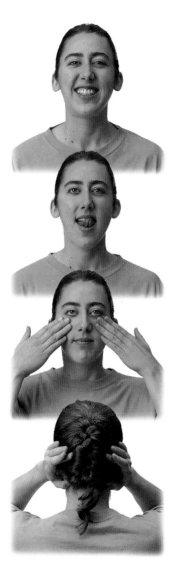

1 Sit upright on a chair or cross-legged on the floor. Tap your teeth together 20–30 times—this increases blood circulation to the gums and helps prevent dental disease. Do not do this if you have gum disease or uneven teeth.

2 Massage the fronts, backs, and sides of your teeth with your tongue tip until you feel a tingling sensation. This helps to encourage healthy gums. It also keeps the mouth clean and increases production of saliva. Swallow at the end of the massage.

3 Rub your hands together to warm the palms. Gently rub them across the cheeks from the nose, from the center of the forehead to the top of the ears, and from the chin to the bottom of the ears. Repeat 20 times. This increases the supply of blood and nutrients to the skin and helps keep it youthful. Do not do this if you have a skin infection.

4 Place your hands on your head so that the base of the palms cover the ears. Cross each index finger over the middle finger of the same hand. Draw them down the back of the head: this works an important acupuncture point that helps to calm and invigorate.

Upper Body Stretch

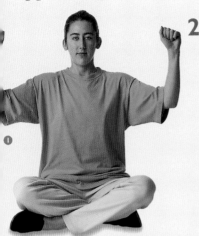

2 Bring your hands together and interlock the fingers. Raise your arms above your head, turning the palms to face upward. Repeat this action up to ten times: it helps to open the chest and encourage good breathing. Keep breathing evenly throughout the exercise.

1 Make loose fists with your hands. Raise them to head level, bending the elbows and keeping the knuckles pointing forward. Lower the forearms, dropping the hands so that the knuckles face downward, and then raise them. Do this up to ten times: it helps to keep the shoulder joints flexible.

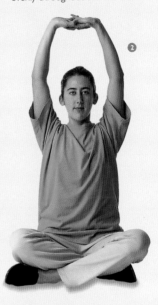

3 Lower the arms to the chest. Curl the last three fingers of the right hand into the palm and point the index finger and thumb upward. Extend the right arm to the side and turn your head to the right. At the same time, make a fist with the left hand and draw it to the left—as if drawing a bow. Then do the same action on the right. Repeat ten times: this opens the chest and works the shoulders.

Toe Touching

Sit on the floor, legs out straight. Bend forward from the waist and catch hold of your knees, shins, or toes—whichever you can manage. Repeat ten times, moving slowly and keeping your back straight. Breathe out as you bend forward and in as you come up. Do not strain, and leave this step out if you cannot easily sit on the floor.

Energizing Self-Massage

Use the last three fingers of your right hand to rub the lower abdomen in a clockwise direction. Do 30 rotations, working slowly. You are rubbing the tan tien— the center of the body's energy in Chinese medicine. This helps to strengthen the internal organs.

2 Rub your hands together to warm the palms. Then place them behind the waist, over the kidneys, as shown below. Rub your hands back and forth about 30 times. This helps to prevent lower back pain and boosts your general sense of well-being.

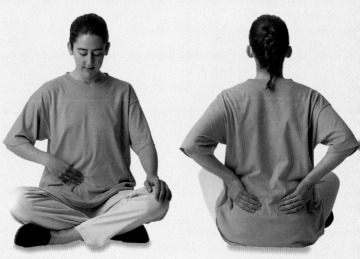

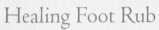

❶ This acupuncture point is powerful, but very safe: it helps to revive the spirits.

Healing Foot Rub

Warm the hands by rubbing the palms together. Use the three middle fingers of your right hand to rub the sole of first your left foot, then the right one. This is deeply relaxing and helps to boost the circulation of the feet. Then use your fingers to gently massage just below the ball, about one-third of the way down the foot. This stimulates a helpful acupuncture point that has a simultaneously reviving and soothing effect.

Foot Treading

Stand tall, with one foot in front of the other. Lift and lower the feet alternately: inhale as you lift and exhale as you place the foot back down. Raise and lower each foot five times, then swap their position and repeat. This helps to work the leg muscles and improves the circulation.

Strength-Building Routine

We tend to lose muscle tone as we grow older. This traditional Chinese routine—known as yi chin ching—is intended to keep the muscles and tendons strong. It was a popular method of fitness in ancient China and is still practiced today. The movements are demanding, so it is suitable only for those who are already reasonably fit. Practice daily, and build your routine slowly: start with the first few exercises and add the others one by one as your flexibility and strength improve. Keep the body in a relaxed position, and make sure that all your movements are slow, controlled, and relaxed.

Starting Position

Stand tall, tucking in your chin and tailbone to keep your spine straight. Keep your head erect and in line with the spine. Your feet should be shoulder-distance apart, facing forward. Let your arms hang down by your sides, keeping a little space under the armpits and letting your palms face backward. Relax the hands and splay the fingers slightly. Relax the shoulders. Breathe evenly for a few moments in this position to relax the body and quieten the mind.

Folding Hands

1 Raise your arms up to shoulder level, letting the backs of the hand lead the movement—your hands should feel almost as if they are floating upward. Keep the palms facing downward.

2 Now bend your elbows and draw the hands toward your chest until the fingers are almost touching. Let the elbows drop downward and keep the shoulders relaxed. Slowly drop the hands back down to the starting position.

Raising Arms

1 Bring your hands out to the sides, turning the palms upward. Keep the elbows slightly bent: they should never be locked straight. As you move the hands, bring more of your weight onto your toes.

2 Lift the arms up to shoulder level, keeping the palms facing upward. Do not tense the shoulders. As you raise the arms, bring all of your weight onto your toes, letting the heels rise off the ground. Lower the arms and heels at the same time.

Supporting the Sky

1 Resume the starting position, standing tall but relaxed, with your arms by your sides and palms facing inward. Move your arms out to the sides and then up above your head, in a large circular motion. Turn your hands so that the palms are facing upward and the tips of your fingers are almost touching—as if you were trying to hold up the sky. As you lift the arms, come onto your toes, letting your heels lift up slightly.

2 Bring your hands into fists—but do not clench them so hard that you feel tension in in the forearms. Lower them to shoulder height, bringing your heels to the ground at the same time. Keep the movement controlled and slow—you should feel the muscles in your arms working.

Exchanging the Stars

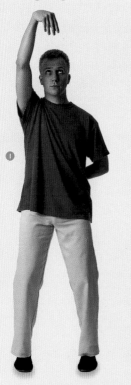

2 Lower your right hand and let it rest on your back, behind the waist. At the same time, raise your left arm above the head, dropping the hand and bringing the fingers closer together. Look up at your hand. Take a few deep, slow breaths in this position. Repeat these arm movements twice more on each side.

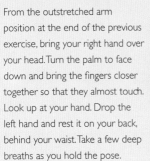

From the outstretched arm position at the end of the previous exercise, bring your right hand over your head. Turn the palm to face down and bring the fingers closer together so that they almost touch. Look up at your hand. Drop the left hand and rest it on your back, behind your waist. Take a few deep breaths as you hold the pose.

> **HELPFUL HINT**
>
> Lift up your head to look at the raised hand, but make sure that you do not tense the muscles of the neck.

Moving the Cow

1 Start from the final position of the previous exercise. Lower the left hand and then bring it back behind your hip, forming a loose fist with the hand. At the same time, take a wide step forward with the right foot, keeping both feet facing in the same direction. Bring the right hand forward and up, curling the fingers so that they just touch—your hand should form a hook shape. Inhale, and pull slightly downward on the right hand—imagine you are pulling a cow's tail. Exhale and focus on the left hand, pushing it slightly forward as if moving the cow on.

2 Drop the right hand behind your hip, bringing it into a fist. Step forward with the left foot, maintaining your wide stance. Raise the left hand above shoulder level, bringing it into a hook shape. Inhale and draw the hand downward. Exhale and push forward with the right fist. You should feel the muscles working in the shoulders, trunk, and legs. Repeat the exercise twice more.

Pushing Palms

2 Exhale and extend the arms in front of you, turning the palms to face outward as shown. Remember to keep a slight bend in the elbows. Keep your back straight as you do this: do not lean forward. Inhale and draw the hands back toward your chest, turning the palms to face downward. Do this movement three times.

1 Starting from the final position of the previous exercise, step forward with the right foot to line up the feet: they should be hip-distance apart. Bring both hands in front of the chest, bending the elbows and turning the palms to face comfortably downward. Check that your shoulders are relaxed, and that your head and spine are erect.

Grounding the Feet

1 Starting from the last posture of the previous sequence, move your left foot to the left, so that your feet are wide apart. Bend your knees and extend your arms out to the your sides, with your hands at shoulder level and palms facing downward.

HELPFUL HINT

As you squat, keep the knees facing in the same direction as your feet and do not allow them to extend over your toes.

2 Squat down, keeping your back straight and head erect. Lower your arms and bring your hands over the thighs with your palms pointing downward. Keep the hands relaxed, with the fingers splayed.

Throwing Fists

1 Starting from the final position of the previous exercise, make loose fists with your hands and turn them so that the knuckles face downward. Lower them to waist level. Then swing the right fist across your body as you turn the waist to the left. At the same time, draw the left fist back, turning the hand upward.

3 Come up from the squat, and raise your hands: turn the palms up and bring the hands in so that the fingers almost touch. Then, turn your hands so that the fingers point forward. Repeat the exercise twice. After the final movement, move the left foot in so that the feet are hip-distance apart again.

2 Now draw the right fist down, turning the hand to face up. Swing the left fist across your body as the palm turns down and you turn the waist to the right. Repeat twice, coordinating your actions into a steady flow.

Stalking Prey like a Cat

1 Starting from the last posture of the previous sequence, drop your hands down. They should be just in front of your body, with your palms facing behind you.

2 Take a long step forward with the right foot, bending the knee and letting the left leg stretch out behind you. Lean forward over the right leg, keeping your back straight, and rest your fingertips (or your palms) on the floor. Keep the head erect.

3 Breathing out, bend your elbows a little more and lean further forward —as if you are a cat stalking its prey. Breathing in, straighten the arms and move back again. Do this forward–backward action twice more. Then come up slowly; you may find it easier to slide the left foot forward first.

4 Now take a long step forward with your left foot, bending the left knee well and letting the right leg straighten behind you. Do the forward–backward action described in step 3 three times.

5 Come up slowly—again, you may find it easier to slide the right foot forward first. Return to the starting position.

HELPFUL HINT

Do not include this exercise in your routine unless you can squat easily. Go only as far as is comfortable for you, and do not arch the back.

195

Bending Forward

1 Take a few deep breaths in the starting position. Check that your shoulders are relaxed, that your chin and tailbone are tucked in, and that your head is erect and in line with the spine. Keep your knees slightly bent.

2 Raise the arms and bring the hands behind the head. Interlink your fingers, and rest the palms at the base of the skull. Move your elbows back so that they extend comfortably out to the sides.

3 Exhaling, bend forward from the waist, going only as far as feels comfortable for you—if you feel strain in the lower back, you have gone too far. While you are in this position, you can practice the following acupressure technique. Unlink your hands, and cross each index finger over the middle finger of the same hand, as shown. Keep the hands on the back of the skull, resting the palms over the base of the ears. Draw your index fingers down to the base of the head— this stimulates an invigorating acupuncture point that also helps relieve headaches and neck stiffness. Do this ten times, then come up slowly as you breathe in. Drop the arms to your sides.

CAUTION
You should not do this exercise if you have high blood pressure.

Touch the Ground, Reach to the Sky

1 Raise your hands to chest height, turning the palms to face outward. Push out, extending your arms out, but keeping a slight bend in the elbows. Keep the back straight and the shoulders relaxed.

2 Draw your hands back toward your chest, bending the elbows so that they extend out to the sides. Interlace your fingers and turn the palms to face downward. Keep breathing steadily throughout.

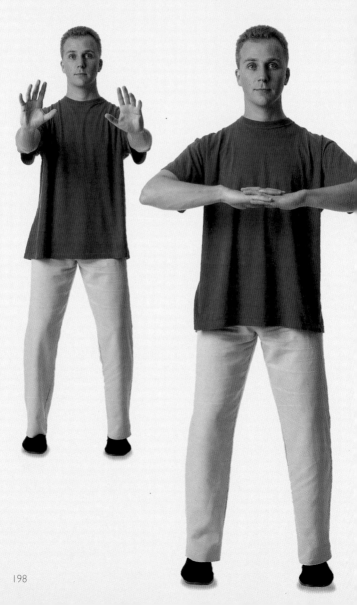

3 Breathing out, bend from the waist. Take your hands as close to the floor as possible, without straining. Don't worry if you cannot bend very far: you will get more flexible with practice. Look just ahead of your hands and breathe evenly.

4 Inhale as you come up slowly. Release your fingers and raise your arms above your head, turning your palms to face upward and bringing the tips of your middle fingers together. At the same time, bring your body weight onto your toes and let the heels lift off the ground.

5 Lower your arms and come back onto your heels. Stand and breathe evenly for a minute to finish.

CAUTION
Do not bend forward if you suffer from high blood pressure.

Glossary

ACUPUNCTURE Complementary therapy in which fine needles are used to restore the flow of energy (chi) within the body, promoting good health. It can be helpful for some musculoskeletal problems, including sciatica and fibromyalgia.

ACUTE Symptom or condition that comes on suddenly and is short-lived.

BONE-DENSITY SCAN Technique in which low-level X-rays are used to measure the density of bone. It is used to confirm a diagnosis of osteoporosis.

CARDIOVASCULAR Relating to the circulation system—the heart and blood vessels.

CERVICAL SPINE The seven bones of the neck.

CHIROPRACTOR Physical therapist who works mainly on the spine, in order to correct misalignments.

CHOLESTEROL A fatty substance in the blood that can block the arteries. A high level of cholesterol in the blood increases the risk of heart disease.

CHRONIC Term used to describe a symptom or condition that is long-lasting and slow to change.

COCCYX The base of the spine, which is also known as the tailbone. It consists of four vertebrae that are fused together.

CT SCAN Computerized tomography scans are a sophisticated form of X-ray that allows cross-sectional pictures of the inside of the body. As with an X-ray, the patient is exposed to a tiny dose of radiation. CT scans are most often used to investigate the brain, abdomen, and spine.

LIGAMENTS Strong bands of fibrous tissue that connect two bones and help to stabilize a joint.

LUMBAR SPINE The five bones of the lower back.

MRI Magnetic resonance imaging is a diagnostic technique that is used to examine soft tissues such as the brain, heart, muscles, and ligaments. The procedure is non-invasive and, unlike X-rays, does not require any exposure to radiation.

NON-STEROIDAL ANTI-INFLAMMATORY DRUGS A group of drugs that have pain-killing and anti-inflammatory effects. They are often used to relieve long-term musculoskeletal disorders, such as arthritis, as well as muscle strain and other short-term problems. They should not be taken by people with asthma or kidney problems.

OSTEOPATH Physical therapist who manipulates the bones and joints to improve alignment and restore normal movement.

PHYSIOTHERAPIST A physical therapist who helps people with bone, joint, and muscle disorders. A variety of techniques are used including specialized exercises, massage, heat, or ultrasound treatment, and hydrotherapy.

PILATES Safe and effective form of body conditioning that emphasizes precise, controlled movements and good breathing technique to tone the muscles and improve posture.

SACRUM Five fused vertebrae in the lower spine. They form a joint with the pelvic bone, called the sacroiliac joint.

TAI CHI Traditional Chinese form of exercise, which works the whole body and involves flowing, controlled movements. It is said to be suitable for people of all ages.

TENDON Strong bands of fibrous tissue that connect muscles to bones, letting movement take place.

THORACIC SPINE The twelve vertebrae in the chest region.

X-RAY Diagnostic imaging technique that uses radiation to produce images of inside the body. X-rays are commonly used to investigate bone problems, particularly fractures, because they are most efficient at providing pictures of dense tissue. X-rays are safe because the dose of radiation used is small and most people have them rarely; however, they are not advised in pregnancy.

YOGA Traditional Indian practice that combines physical exercises and breathing techniques to improve flexibility and strength.

Further Reading

RICHARD BRENNAN, *The Alexander Technique Manual: A Step-by-Step Guide to Improve Breathing, Posture and Wellbeing*, Little, Brown, 1999.

DR ANTHONY CAMPBELL, *Back: Your 100 Questions Answered*, Newleaf, 2001

LEON CHAITOW *Arthritis*, Thorsons, 1998

EDWARD C. CHANG (TRANSLATOR), *Knocking at the Gate of Life: Healing Exercises from the Official Manual of the People's Republic of China*, Laurel Glen, 2000

KIM DAVIES, *The Tai Chi Directory*, Newleaf, 2004

JOE ELLIS, JOE HENDERSON, *Running Injury-Free: How to Prevent, Treat and Recover from Dozens of Painful Problems*, Rodale, 1994

DEBORAH AND SIMON FIELDING,. *The Healthy Back Exercise Book*, Ted Smart, 2001

RONALD MELZACK AND PATRICK WALL, *The Challenge of Pain*, Penguin Books, 1996

LYNNE ROBINSON, *The Body Control Back Book*, Pan, 2002

DR CAROLINE SHREEVE, *Bones: Your 100 Questions Answered*, Newleaf, 2001

TONY SMITH, *BMA Family Doctor Series: Osteoporosis*, Dorling Kindersley, 1999

DAVA SOBELL AND ARTHUR C. KLEIN, *Arthritis: The Complete Guide to Relief Using Methods That Really Work*, Constable, 1998

STELLA WELLAR, *The Yoga Back Book: The Gentle Yet Effective Way to Spinal Health*, HarperCollins, 2000

WILLIAM WEINTRAUB ET AL, *Tendon and Ligament Healing: A New Approach to Sports and Overuse Injury*, Paradigm Publications, 2003

Osteoporosis: Causes, Prevention and Treatment, National Osteoporosis Society, 1999

Understanding Back Trouble, A Consumer Publication, Which? Books, 1991

Useful Addresses

United Kingdom

ARTHRITIS CARE
18 Stephenson Way,
London NW1 2HD
Telephone: 020 7380 6500
www.arthritiscare.org.uk

BACKCARE
16 Elmtree Rd, Teddington,
Middlesex TW11 BST
Telephone: 020 8977 5474
www.backcare.org

BRITISH MASSAGE THERAPY COUNCIL
17 Rymers Lane, Oxford OX4 3JU
Telephone: 01865 774123
www.btmc.co.uk

GENERAL CHIROPRACTIC COUNCIL
344–354 Gray's Inn Rd,
London W4 1PP
Telephone: 020 8742 2605
www.gcc-uk.org

GENERAL OSTEOPATHIC COUNCIL,
Osteopathy House, 176 Tower
Bridge Rd, London SE1 3LU.
Telephone: 020 7357 6655
www.osteopathy.org.uk

NATIONAL OSTEOPOROSIS SOCIETY
PO Box 10, Radstock,
Bath BA3 3YB
Telephone: 01761 471771
www.nos.org.uk

United States

AMERICAN CHIROPRACTIC
ASSOCIATION
1701 Clarendon Blvd, Arlington,
VA 22209.
Telephone: 703 276 8800
www.amerchiro.org

AMERICAN OSTEOPATHIC
ASSOCIATION
142 East Ohio Street, Chicago,
IL 60611
Telephone: 312 761 2682
www.aoa-net.org

AMERICAN MASSAGE THERAPY
ASSOCIATION
1701 820 Davis Street, Suite 100,
Evanston, IL 60611
Telephone: 312 761 2682
www.amtamassage.org

ARTHRITIS FOUNDATION
PO Box 7669, Atlanta,
GA 30357-0669
Telephone: 1-800-283-7800
www.arthritis.org

NATIONAL OSTEOPOROSIS
FOUNDATION
1232 22nd Street NW
Washington, DC 20037-1292
Telephone: 202-223-2226
www.nof.org

Index

Acknowledgments

Special thanks go to Jonathan Bastable
for his pithy comments on the text, and to Juliet Cox
for her advice on acupuncture.

Picture credits

Photographs

Corbis 6 (the dancer), 16 (the violin
player), 168 (the women exercising),
174 (the couple sleeping)

Illustrations

Michael Courtney 8, 11, 13, 15, 21,
27, 48, 49, 50, 51, 53, 54, 55, 57, 59,
80, 90, 91, 92, 93, 94, 95, 96, 97, 109,
110, 111, 113, 114, 117, 157, 158, 159

Guy Smith 9, 16, 17, 82, 85, 103, 143,
165, 200, 203, 204, 207, 208